Praise for *Side by Side*

Side by Side is beautifully written, heartfelt, and profound. The authors traveled the country to interview older couples about their marriages. Their questions were excellent and the couples they interviewed answered in honest, articulate, and detailed ways. The stories they tell are powerful and poignant teaching stories. The couples were from diverse backgrounds and parts of the country, but they shared many common traits. All were spiritual seekers striving for deep and mutually satisfying relationships. Even as they said goodbye to parents and approached their own deaths, they also faced a world in crisis. In the last chapter, the authors share their own marital struggles. I greatly respected their candor and commitment to each other. All older people now face the loss of the world as we knew it. These stories of marriages can help us understand how to face even the greatest challenges with love, joy, and equanimity.

MARY PIPHER AUTHOR OF *A LIFE IN LIGHT* AND *WOMEN ROWING NORTH*

We're all just walking each other home," said Ram Dass. Here's a book rich with insights into how aging couples in committed relationships are making that walk in ways that help them find wholeness. For several months, Caryl and Jay Casbon traveled the country interviewing couples about the relational dance where we sometimes step on each other's toes and sometimes sweep each other off our feet, learning how to move to the music that makes each other's heart beat. The result is a book of honest and heartfelt conversations from which there is much to learn about the ups and downs of intimate love as a vale of soul-making.

SHARON PALMER & PARKER J. PALMER AUTHOR OF *LET YOUR LIFE SPEAK* AND *THE COURAGE TO TEACH*

It seems like just yesterday that I was reading books on how to prepare for marriage. Then I read a pile of books to help with communication, parenting, budgeting, conflict resolution, time management . . . the challenges of a marriage in motion. And suddenly now, I find a beautiful book for aging couples . . . just what I need now. *Side by Side* unfolds like an adventure and leaves you with so much to think about, individually and together, and so much to live into each irreplaceable day. It even includes abundant resources to use the book in small groups. Highly recommended!

BRIAN D. MCLAREN AUTHOR OF *FAITH AFTER DOUBT*

As someone trying to nurture a marriage in mid-life, I found this book so rare, comforting, and revelatory. Finally, real couples talking about the struggles with our shadows, our family of origin conditioning, and the beast of logistics, while also painting a picture of the sacred work of showing up for someone you love, the physical closeness unlike anything else, the shared adoration for kids and community. *Side by Side* helped me take the long view—a real gift at this moment in my own journey.

COURTNEY E. MARTIN AUTHOR OF *LEARNING IN PUBLIC* AND *THE EXAMINED FAMILY* NEWSLETTER

Each couple's soul story offers pearls of wisdom informed by age and experience. The Readers' Guide is such a thoughtful gift to help us explore our own journey as we step together into this new phase of life.

HELEN DAVIDSON BLOGGER AND LIFE-STORY FACILITATOR FOR OLDER WOMEN AT AGELESSPOSSIBILITIES.ORG

As an Episcopal priest, I frequently work with couples preparing to be married. Their focus is, understandably, on the upcoming wedding and the beginnings of their new life together. Although *Side by Side* focuses on aging couples, still the wisdom of this book, and the stories shared, offer so much for couples at any stage in their relationship, even those just beginning their marriage journey. Embracing the adage, "begin as you mean to go on," *Side by Side* should become required reading for every new couple I meet with.

THE REV. ELIZABETH MOLITORS   RECTOR, TRINITY EPISCOPAL CHURCH, SANTA BARBARA, CALIFORNIA

The Casbons show us how beautiful healing can happen when soulmates show up fully to support each other's spiritual growth. Thanks to these wise couples, we can all learn more about walking the path of Love amidst the mundane and meaningful challenges of partnerships, aging, and simply being human.

CHRISTINE LOVE-MACLEOD & AINSLIE MACLEOD
AUTHOR OF THE INSTRUCTION AND THE OLD SOUL'S GUIDEBOOK

Side by Side shares moving stories about couples who see relationship as well as aging as paths for spiritual growth and who dance with the gifts and challenges of sacred relationship.

HEATHER ENSWORTH PHD   AUTHOR OF *FINDING OUR CENTER* AND CO-AUTHOR OF *FROM TRAUMA TO HEALING*

What makes one marriage last and others fail? This book can help answer that question. The guidance and knowledge of thirteen couples tell their story and offer their age-old wisdom on how they learned to adapt and conquer obstacles that threatened to tear them apart. *Side by Side: The Sacred Art of Couples Aging with Wisdom & Love* is a fascinating reading experience. It made me stop and realize the problems couples face together and how they can keep their love still strong and shining bright. Caryl & Jay Casbon are two talented authors. There was never a moment that I found myself bored reading this book. Instead, I eagerly awaited the next chapter to discover another couple's story. This book would make a wonderful wedding present for all young couples. The wisdom it contains could help them.

MIDWEST BOOK REVIEW

CARYL & JAY CASBON

SIDE by SIDE

the sacred art of couples aging
with wisdom & love

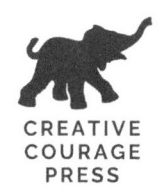

CREATIVE
COURAGE
PRESS

Copyright © 2023 by Caryl & Jay Casbon
All rights reserved. No part of this publication may be reproduced, distributed, or transmitted in form without permission other than for review purposes without written permission of the publisher. Contact the publisher to request reprints, permissions, quantity discounts, and special editions for educational and organizational use.

Creative Courage Press (Palisade, CO) | www.CreativeCouragePress.com
(970) 812-3224 | hello@creativecouragepress.com

First edition (all formats): 2023

Library of Congress Cataloging-in-Publication Data
    Names: Casbon, Caryl, author. | Casbon, Jay, author.
    Title: Side by side : the sacred art of couples aging with wisdom & love / Caryl and Jay Casbon.
    Description: Includes bibliographical references. | Palisade, CO: Creative Courage Press, 2023.
    Identifiers: LCCN: 2023909195 | ISBN: ISBN 978-1-959-92104-2 (print) | 978-1-959-92105-9 (ebook)
    Subjects: LCSH Marital quality. | Marriage. | Older couples. | Married people—Religious life. | Spirituality. | Older people—Psychology. | Love in old age. | BISAC FAMILY & RELATIONSHIPS / Marriage & Long-Term Relationships | SELF-HELP / Aging | RELIGION / Spirituality
    Classification: LCC HQ734 .C37 2023 | DDC 306.81—dc23

Neither the publisher nor the authors shall be held liable or responsible for any loss, actions, or damage allegedly arising from any suggestion or information contained in this book. This book explores themes about committed relationships and ways to "enlighten" them through deep, soulful sharing. It is not intended as a substitute for therapy.

The Circle of Trust® approach is a registered trademark of the Center for Courage & Renewal.
Godly Play® is a registered trademark of the Godly Play Foundation.

Cover art and interior art copyright © 2023 Karen Rauppius
Cover and interior design: Karen Polaski
Editor: Shelly Francis. Editing Intern: Annalyse Hambleton
Proofreader: Rebecca Job
Author photo: Dave Hoffman

For the couples who generously opened their homes
and hearts to us and shared the gift of their stories
which serve as the foundation for this book.

For our therapist, Thery Jenkins, and the other often
unsung healers, therapists, coaches, and spiritual directors
who are committed to helping couples grow stronger, side
by side, as they age together with Spirit, wisdom, and love.

*Beautiful young people are accidents of nature,
but beautiful old people are works of art.*

ELEANOR ROOSEVELT

CONTENTS

INTRODUCTION Inspirited by a
Dream: The Story Behind *Side by Side* — 1

Beatitudes for Couples — 10

1 Blessed Is the Couple Who Welcomes Divine
Presence into Their Midst   JIM & MARIANNE HOUSTON — 13

2 Blessed Is the Couple Who Embraces
All Seasons of Life   CARYL & JEFF CRESWELL — 29

3 Blessed Is the Couple Who Welcomes
the Stranger   LAURIE RUTENBERG & GARY SCHOENBERG — 45

4 Blessed Is the Couple Who Confronts
Their Own Shadows   PAUL & ROZ DUMESNIL — 65

5 Blessed Is the Couple Who Listens Deeply
to Each Other   STEVE & FAYE ORTON SNYDER — 79

6 Blessed Is the Couple Who Practices
Compassion   BOBBY BELLAMY & BARBARA BLAIN-BELLAMY — 93

7 Blessed Is the Couple Who Enjoys the
Fruits of Mutuality   SALLY HARE & JIM ROGERS — 111

8 Blessed Is the Couple Who Extends
Tender Care When Suffering   ANNE & TOM BUTLER — 127

9 Blessed Is the Couple Who Recognizes the Indwelling
  Spirit in All of Life PATSY GRACE & HARVEY BOTTELSEN   141

10 Blessed Is the Couple Who Dances with the
   Tension Between "Me" & "We" RICK & MARCY JACKSON   155

11 Blessed Is the Couple Who Practices
   the Sabbath KAREN NOORDHOFF & DAVID HAGSTROM   169

12 Blessed Is the Couple Who Extends
   Mercy & Forgiveness MICHAEL & EILEEN HEATON   185

13 Blessed Is the Couple Who Offers Beneficial Presence
   Across the Generations RUTH SHAGOURY & JIM WHITNEY   201

   CONCLUSION Lessons from the Road to *Side by Side*   215

   Acknowledgments   229

   APPENDIX I Interview Questions
   for the *Side by Side* Project   231

   APPENDIX II Touchstones for Couples' Group Work   237

   READERS' GUIDE Exploring the
   Stories & Themes in *Side by Side*   241

   Notes   271
   About the Authors   275
   About Creative Courage Press   277

SIDE by SIDE

To journey without being changed is to be a nomad. To change without journeying is to be a chameleon. To journey and to be transformed by the journey is to be a pilgrim.

MARK NEPO

INTRODUCTION

Inspirited by a Dream: The Story Behind *Side by Side*

ONE MORNING I awoke to discover Jay waiting for me, wide-eyed and eager to share an idea that came to him in a dream. This was a numinous dream, coming from Spirit, charging us to interview aging couples in committed relationships living into the winter season of their lives. A title popped into my head, and I blurted out, "Jay, I think I know what we can call this project: *Side by Side*." It stuck and became our north star. We would film older couples, interweaving a trinity of themes: relationships, aging, and spirituality. And then we would find a way to share what we learned with as many people as possible. Game on.

To be clear, while we focus on spirituality, we recognize that couples approach the Great Mystery and their search for meaning in myriad ways, such as spending time in nature, working for social justice, practicing meditation, privately studying poetry and sacred texts, and so on. Many couples are "unchurched" and don't participate in organized religion but have crafted and honed their own unique ways of practicing and sharing their spiritual journeys as a cornerstone for their relationship. We embrace, as the title states, the notion of committed relationships as "sacred art," which we hope will become clear in meaning as you read the stories in this book. *Side by Side* is also for couples who may not have named their spiritual journey as vital but are curious to see how other couples are doing so.

This dream found us both in the midst of befriending our own aging along with one of life's more disorienting initiations: retirement. At heart, we were worker bees and sincerely enjoyed our careers in education and ministry; this wasn't an easy change. We were not looking for another job either, yet this *Side by Side* dream, what we have come to understand now as a "commission," arrived right when we had the time to pursue it. It foreshadowed a theme that often occurred in the interviews: retirement doesn't mean that your soul's callings fall silent. Instead, it is an invitation for re-formation, allowing one's old life to recede and making room for new priorities. Now free from "making a living," we began to consider "making a life." *Side by Side* transformed from a dream fragment to a full-blown adventure that has consumed us ever since.

We purchased a Winnebago and named it *The Dharma Dog* to pursue the dream. "Dharma" translates as one's destiny, a sacred path or duty. A dog, well, follows its nose and knows a good bone when it whiffs one. That, in essence, describes our research methods. Driving across the country and back in two months, over 8,000 miles, we dodged hurricanes and camped among the buffalo in Yellowstone and the iguanas, sandhill cranes, and wild pigs in Florida. The journey enabled us to arrange three-day visits with the couples and carry with us our shelter, camera equipment, and rescue dog, Lily Rose, who showed up at our doorstep one day before we departed.

"Naivete is the mother of adventure"[1] is quoted on the first page of a true story about Rinker Buck, a brave fellow inspired to travel the Oregon Trail in a covered wagon, re-creating the conditions of the original pioneers as much as possible. Temperamental mules, fractured wagon wheels, lousy weather, and numerous other near-disasters not imagined when he guilelessly set forth plagued his journey. The disasters also dished up the memorable guts of his narrative, where his character and skills were tested. His journey serves as a metaphor for our project. Jay and I also headed down the *Side by Side* trail, profoundly naïve regarding what it would ask of us, where it would take us, and what disasters (like a pandemic) would impede our progress. The journey presented a much wilder, more difficult, and heartwarming odyssey than we could have imagined. At times, it became a grueling, heartbreaking ordeal. We began to say, "We are not doing this project but undergoing it."

Anyone who has traveled in an RV understands what its cramped confines, daily moving on to explore unknown territory, and its tendency to break down (like the prominent crack in our windshield that funneled an internal waterfall onto the dashboard during torrential rainstorms in North Dakota), do to your relationship. It brings out your best and worst qualities. For us, the RV stands as another metaphor for the conditions aging couples face: lots of time in the smaller world of your home, unpredictable weather conditions, unexpected delays and repairs with health problems, changing status, and freedom to go where you want to go. Jay and I witnessed each other's tenacious strengths when tested under adversity and learned to be gentle when we got tired at the end of the day—or reactive amidst troubles. Filming, traveling, and writing together intensified the conditions in the cauldron of our marriage, which became an unintended but necessary part of the story.

The Oregon-bound pioneers traversed dirt roads littered with discarded tables, bureaus, and other family heirlooms their fellow travelers thought they could not leave home without. They quickly discovered that the weight and bulk of their possessions endangered their progress, burdened their mules, and broke down their fragile wagons. We, too, had to cast away treasured ideas of what we thought was necessary when we began. For instance, during the first year of the pandemic, right when we had completed the interviews, we wrote a long, wordy draft of an entirely different book than you see here. Our friend and now publisher/editor, Shelly Francis, informed us that we missed the mark and needed to rewrite the book in a story format. So, we "tossed the first draft off the wagon," leaving behind a year of work. The second version is what you hold in your hands, with chapters highlighting each couple's story. Also, amidst the rewrite, Jay and I ran into serious relationship concerns after twenty years of marriage. We found a therapist, stopped writing for a while, and delved into our dynamics. I underwent a total hip replacement and didn't write a word for two months while I healed.

At the time, all of these challenges felt like roadblocks or, at best, significant detours. In truth, they resulted in what we hope is a much-improved book and significant growth in our relationship. Our callings take us into the territory of our soul's inner work. Our souls don't give a rip about deadlines or even the finished product; they want us to grow. Troubles have a way of attracting grace and guidance in dark places, offering what we most need. This is good news for those of us aging and doing the hard work of relationships.

We are often asked, "How did you select the couples?" The quick answer is we turned to people we considered "old souls" living in committed relationships with spiritual practices embedded in their daily lives. We sought couples capable of vulnerability in front of others and willing to "go public" by discussing the project's themes in front of a camera: aging, relationships, and spirituality—not an easy ask. Half of the couples we approached said no. For some, it was too exposed; others were insecure about the health of their relationship. For the gay couples we approached, it was simply too public. We truly understood. This project reflects some of the challenges, wisdom, and stories of this generation of elders. It does not include some of the rich diversity of faiths, sexual orientations, races, and cultures living in this country today. It is simply a snapshot in time of thirteen couples interviewed before the pandemic.

We wanted soul stories. There is a significant difference between soul stories versus ego or hero stories.[2] We all tell ego stories—the ones recounted for self-promotion—that highlight achievements and successes and are designed to manage a controlled image or persona. There is a place and time for ego stories, as when applying for a job. But soul stories, much like Rinker Buck's Oregon Trail yarns, include ambiguous endings, complexity, beauty, and darkness. They aren't recounted to promote the ego or make us look good but to explore the truth. Soul stories honor vulnerable encounters with failure as well as achievements. They include emotions often hidden from sight and rejected by society, like fear, shame, passion, and anger. The experience of aging, as well as intimate relationships, belongs to the geography of the soul.

As Jay and I retired, we wondered about our relationship as we grow older together. What does love mean now, at this age? How much time together is a good thing? How do we honor our natural leanings toward more solitude, interiority, creativity, and spiritual growth? What can we give back to our troubled world? Who will die first, and how will the survivor bear it? How can we make the most out of these remaining years?

It is a rare privilege to have access to another couple's world. Couples are seldom witnessed; following the fanfare of the wedding, they retreat to the privacy of their homes, mostly sheltered from others' gazes. We have never experienced anything quite like staying with a couple over two to three days, preparing meals and taking walks, then diving into structured, in-depth conversations, asking set questions, and listening to their responses over six hours of filming. Each time, we entered a sacred space. By the end of the interview, we felt in awe as well as deep love for the couple, without exception. And we didn't want to leave. We discovered a great nobility in this generation of aging couples.

The couples, in turn, often thanked us for the chance to reflect on their lives and history, to hear what the other had to say, and for being witnessed. It was one of the most satisfying experiences of our lives.

It is a secret hidden in plain sight: relationships are hard. Relationships bring us to the edges of endurance, mirror our tragic flaws, shadows, and goodness, and offer the most humbling, fertile path to growth we know of.

We created questions (listed in appendix I) that invited stories of struggles, conflict, love, parents' deaths, mystical experiences and spiritual growth, joy, purpose, and meaning. We drew heavily on our friendships from our community through the Center for Courage & Renewal. For over twenty-five years, Jay and I have worked with many colleagues leading soul-centered, inner-work retreats for teachers, spiritual leaders, and executives, using Quaker practices and the Circle of Trust approach based on the work of author, educator, and activist Parker J. Palmer. These couples were natural for our project.

Some of the couples we found through friends. When someone said to us, "You need to meet these folks," we treated it like a bone on the trail and followed up with their suggestion; many of those connections worked out as well. We made the path by walking and listening to leads, synchronicity, and guidance, and were seldom disappointed.

We hope the use of the story format—the ancient way of passing along history and meaning—captures the unique lessons each couple embodies through their lived experiences. Each of us finds different meanings in stories, and while we share some of our interpretations, we trust you to discover your own.

Our fear now is that we can't do justice to the outpouring of humor, insight, and wisdom the couples shared with us. We have done our imperfect best, we hope.

HOW TO USE THIS BOOK

This book is created for couples interested in consciously walking side by side, making the most of this time of life with the time they have left—to age together as they distill their life experiences, adjusting to the inevitable changes that aging brings. We all learn differently. While you are welcome to read *Side by Side* alone or skip to the chapters that interest you, the reading of it is also intended to be shared in order to create opportunities for dialogue with others. If you are in a committed relationship, we suggest that you set aside time to read this book aloud to each other at your own pace. To get the most out of it, go to the Readers' Guide included at the end of the book. It includes questions and practices designed to initiate discussions on the themes contained in each chapter. If you wish to set up a couples' group, the guide also suggests how to do so.

Additional group work materials, video clips, and support for forming groups will be available on our website as well: www.sidebysideaging.com.

HOW THE BOOK IS STRUCTURED: THE BEATITUDES FOR COUPLES

Side by Side offers a chapter dedicated to telling the story of each of the couples we interviewed, and each chapter begins with a "beatitude." When we traveled to Israel several years ago, we made our way to the Mount of Beatitudes, a hill on the Korazim Plateau by the Sea of Galilee, where many believe Jesus delivered "The Sermon on the Mount," a homily that sheds light on how to live and embody one's faith. The Beatitudes, a part of this sermon, found in the gospel of Mark in the Bible, form an elegant progression of eight blessings and teachings that became a lasting contribution to wisdom literature. Jesus' ministry was never about beliefs but the daily living of spiritual principles to honor and love one another and to practice peace and nonviolence. The Beatitudes' perennial wisdom has inspired work for social justice in society and offered comfort to the suffering.

As we wrote the following chapters, the "Beatitudes for Couples" quietly and organically emerged through the stories. Inspired, we crafted a list of our own "be-attitudes" or blessings that would support the sacred art of messy, challenging, committed relationships. We organized this book around these new Beatitudes for Couples, which informed the chapter titles. A few of these beatitudes are not assigned to one specific couple yet are reflected through many of their stories.

You can find them in their entirety on the following page and as a printable download at our website. While this book is non-denominational, we believe the original Beatitudes and the Beatitudes for Couples are meant to speak to your heart and soul no matter what faith tradition you follow (or none at all).

We have been changed by this journey with the *Side by Side* couples. Our sincere desire is that you may be transformed by their stories as well as you age together, side by side with wisdom and love.

A note about authorship: While we conceived this book and project together, and both interviewed the couples and then transcribed the interviews, Caryl has penned the stories in this book, as we found it challenging to blend our writing styles. Jay focused on the summary of findings, created the Beatitudes for Couples, and consulted with Caryl regularly concerning the themes and content of each chapter. We are thought partners in every aspect of this body of work.

> With blessings and gratitude,
> Caryl & Jay Casbon
> Santa Barbara, California

The Beatitudes for Couples

Blessed is the couple who welcomes Divine
Presence into their midst, for they shall know
Eternal Belonging, grace, and love.

Blessed is the couple who embraces all seasons of
life—the perennial cycles of spring, summer, autumn,
and winter—for they shall know wholeness.

Blessed is the couple who welcomes the stranger
in each other, for they shall find wonder and
encouragement on their growing edges.

Blessed is the couple who confronts their own shadows,
for they shall be freed from blame and projection.

Blessed is the couple who listens deeply to each
other, for they shall be seen, understood, and met.

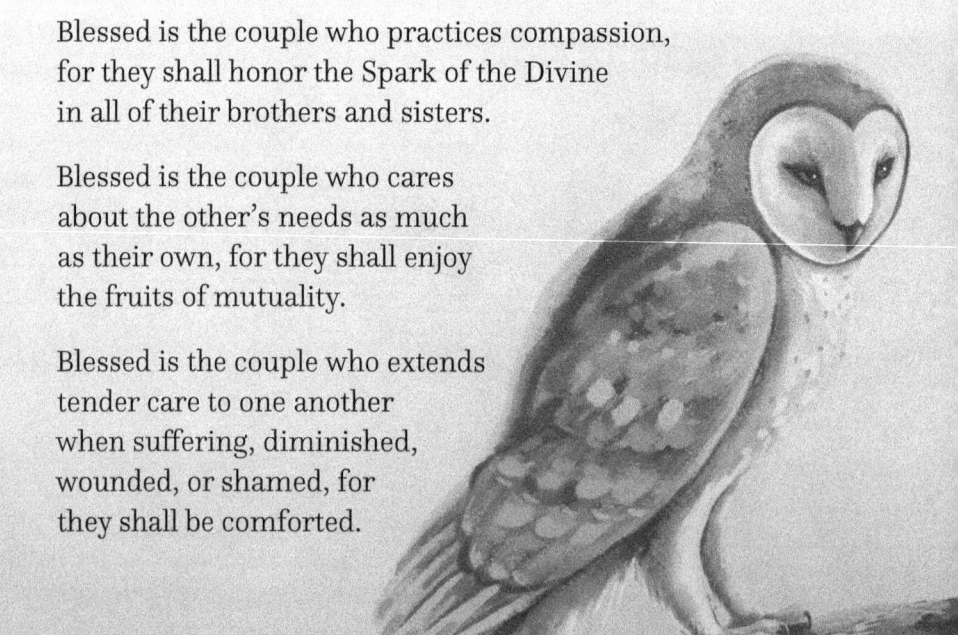

Blessed is the couple who practices compassion,
for they shall honor the Spark of the Divine
in all of their brothers and sisters.

Blessed is the couple who cares
about the other's needs as much
as their own, for they shall enjoy
the fruits of mutuality.

Blessed is the couple who extends
tender care to one another
when suffering, diminished,
wounded, or shamed, for
they shall be comforted.

Blessed is the couple who recognizes the Indwelling Spirit in all of life, for they shall encounter the Mystery and see the Light in all beings.

Blessed is the couple who dances with the tension between "me" and "we," for they shall know companioning without loss of self.

Blessed is the couple who openly and humbly addresses conflict, for they shall find truth, reconciliation, and freedom from violence.

Blessed is the couple who practices Sabbath through the daily bread of devotion, mindfulness, and prayer, for they shall find Home.

Blessed is the couple who extends mercy and forgiveness, for they shall be relieved of resentment and harsh judgment.

Blessed is the couple who offers beneficial presence across the generations, for they shall leave a legacy of love.

Blessed is the couple who celebrates life with the Spirits of tomfoolery, shenanigans, creativity, and play, for they shall know humor and mirth, and have some really good times.

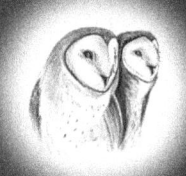

Blessed is the couple who
welcomes Divine Presence into
their midst, for they shall know
Eternal Belonging, grace, and love.

BLESSED IS THE COUPLE WHO
Welcomes Divine Presence into Their Midst

INTRODUCING
JIM & MARIANNE HOUSTON

WHEN WE ENTERED Marianne and Jim Houston's home in Kalamazoo, Michigan, we passed through a hallway that also serves as a gallery. On the right wall are photographs of Jim's entire African American Baptist family, going back to the slave period before the Thirteenth, Fourteenth, and Fifteenth Amendments of the US Constitution. His family photos face Marianne's pictures of her Polish-Catholic clan, gazing back at Jim's. Also adorning the walls are the children's and grandchildren's images, the progeny of their family tree. Among those photographs lives a couple held together by love and history, who treasure every bit of their heritage while honestly acknowledging the struggles of bringing two cultures together. Their peaceful countenance and sparkling eyes tell a story of belonging; Jim and Marianne chose to marry in 1968 when interracial marriage was newly legalized in the US, bravely leaning into a marriage that broke with conventions of the time.

In the den is a photograph of Marianne as a young Catholic novice in full habit, posing with a group of nuns in France in the early 1960s. In this image, Marianne's smile is like the expression of Mona Lisa; a knowing observer can spot a joyful rascal and a genuine original. We were intrigued to learn how Marianne changed from a Sister of Loretto to becoming a married partner of Jim Houston for fifty-one years!

When we asked them what brought them together, we soon discovered the answer. In Marianne's words, "Well, Jim and I met when I was working at the University of Wisconsin in Madison. It was 1967, and as an Air Force sergeant at the base, he was helping to close it down at the time. He was also taking classes and stopped at a coffee house on campus. I walked in, and he saw my girlfriend and me and asked to join us. I said, 'Of course!' That was the beginning of our 52-year relationship. I saw someone kind, smart, funny, and different from the other men I had been dating. I thought, 'What a good new friend,' and that is how it came to me that night."

Jim chimed in. "That is her version. I saw a knockout gal that came in the door and thought, 'What an attractive young lady. I need to know her.' We talked for a half-hour, and I had to go back to the base. I told my buddy right then that I was going to marry her. We got together and began to go out. In little over a year, we dated off and on and then married. There was something about her. I knew she was the one, but I had to convince her. Then I was transferred to Tacoma, where I spent my last two years of enlistment and our first two years of marriage. We then returned to Madison and finally moved to Kalamazoo in 1970 to finish my university studies. We have lived here ever since, where we have become immersed in this community, had our two sons, now grown, and now six grandchildren."

Marianne acknowledged their age difference with humor. "We feel very fortunate. When I met Jim, I was thirty-two, Jim was twenty-three, and I had been a nun from ages eighteen to thirty. I thought I was thirty going on twenty. Jim had been around a little, so I thought he was twenty-three going on thirty-one."

Marianne recalled being recruited to become a secretary for campus police after a young coed was murdered on the UW campus. "I agreed to do that. It was terrifying. Jim knew how I was responding to this and picked me up each morning, so I wouldn't have to walk alone. He came by in the afternoon and escorted me home. I knew that gentlemanly behavior was rare. There are so many examples of that. If I called him, he was there. If I needed him, he was there. And I was there for him. Jim's deepest modus operandi is one of kindness. When I watch him interacting with others, I learn so much about loving-kindness. And his loyalty; I have known since we have been together that he was always there. And besides, he is funny and fun to be with, even when we are upset with each other."

Since Jim and Marianne bring together two different religious and racial traditions, as well as age disparities, we were interested in how this impacted them. When a couple comes together, they always join the two cultures from their respective families of origin, including unspoken rules of communication, expectations, and roles. Starting with their religious backgrounds, they noted that their Roman Catholic and Baptist traditions were "the least of our problems," for they have a mutual understanding of the Christian message and ways of being in the world. They believe that there is only one God. Jim converted to Catholicism but also kept his Baptist roots. They were married in a ceremony with both a Catholic priest and a Protestant minister, and on their fiftieth anniversary, they again celebrated their relationship with both traditions represented.

"I never insisted that he convert," Marianne stated. "I thought he was the best Christian I knew, but with Jamie, our oldest son, Jim thought he should see us practicing a shared tradition. Father Fitz said to Jim, 'I don't know what to do, for you are already baptized. But I can confirm you.' Then Jim replied, 'There is only one thing. I don't do this confession thing. I talk to God with a direct line.' Father Fitz concurred and said, 'I can understand that. I just want to ask you a couple of things. All of our lives, we do things we regret, hurt people, etc., so I am sure you have had things like that in your life.' Then he said, 'I absolve you.'"

Jim added, "That was my one and only confession."

While a mutual acceptance of their religious backgrounds was easily navigated, some of the variations in their family cultures were more challenging. Jim began, "I come from a family that is extremely loud. We are not past the point of coming down on someone who needs it, either. Marianne has had to adjust to people speaking up like this and speaking to someone who needs a comeuppance. I had to get used to her quiet, indirect family, and she, our loudness."

Marianne added, "In my family, we might see a sister do something that bothers us, complain about her behind her back, but not say to her, 'Shut up.' Jim's way of joking is something they do in his culture, which they call 'signify,' what you do with your best friends. They hit their most sensitive areas as a part of a joke. That type of humor was not part of my experience. It is only funny if it is funny for the other person, but not if the other is hurt."

Jim explained, "It is part of my culture from slavery time. How you get through the pain is by laughing. To do otherwise, I've come to learn as a sociologist, would destroy you.

Signifying is a survival mechanism, in addition to laughing, joking, and singing together. I've learned since how the people in the Holocaust survived in the camps. They have discovered some of the most beautiful music written in the camps. There is a lot of comedy displayed by Jewish people that comes out of their pain and suffering. Blacks use humor, music, and laughter as ways to survive."

Marianne noted, "I have come to love it most of the time. And Jim has had to adjust to my seriousness. I tend to take seriously things that he can brush off. I have come to understand that within Jim, his family, and many of our other friends, he can laugh at things, and I say to myself, 'That is not funny. It is hurtful.' Jim says, 'I laugh to keep from crying.'" Marianne concluded, "I've had to adjust to what doesn't seem funny."

Other cultural differences manifested in their approaches to raising their children. Jim came from a strict, authoritarian family, and when we asked about what has tested their relationship, they named this issue. "There was a difference in how we raised our sons," Marianne said. "I was not so focused on being hard on and physical with the boys in terms of spanking. My way wasn't that way, and not my family's way. We had to come to an agreement about that. That is not to say Jim was a tyrant or cruel, but he employed an authoritarian approach to discipline, which we had to talk out. That was a test."

Jim explained his approach to parenting. "Raising our sons, I was not the buddy-buddy type. My message to them was, 'I am not your friend. I am your father.' I don't know if that was right or wrong, but I valued that our sons respected us as elders, here to guide them. That is how I was raised. Now that they are grown, I can be a parent and a friend. There is a little of that which still lingers in me. Each has its value.

In young people today, disrespect is rampant. I know why I was raised to respect elders, and I believe levels of respect need to be maintained. I was raised that kids address elders by their last names. I did not have the right to use their first name. We still address them that way, Mr. So-and-So. There is something good about that. Did my parents ever consider us peers? I am not sure. Yet both of my sons have said to me, 'I am glad you were hard on us. We see our peers and what weaklings they are, and I am glad my dad was hard on me.' During the '70s, some parents were afraid to discipline their children because they thought the children would no longer love them or be afraid of them."

Jim and Marianne also noted that we are now facing several generations raised without fathers in the home. They believe the absence of fathers for the sons has been instrumental in creating violence and anger in young lives.

Most couples also negotiate differences in their personalities. We asked each couple in our interviews what they thought was most difficult about their temperament for their partner. You know, that quality that defies changing and that pushes your buttons. Marianne blurted out a common yet challenging difference. "I am a terminal extrovert. I talk as I think." For many couples, one is an extrovert and the other an introvert. This profoundly impacts communication styles, how much alone time you need, and if you like to think aloud or silently. It is critical to how we approach and process life.

Marianne continued, "I was born with what is today described as hyperactivity, on top of being an ecstatic person. That has been there since I was a child. The earliest thing I can remember my mother saying was, 'Marianne, just be quiet.' Language is both internal and external. What is internal shoots right out of my mouth. It creates a real challenge for me as a facilitator and teacher to be quiet enough to hear my students, I mean, really hear them. My years in the Loretto community, with so much silence, were perfect for me. In my teens and twenties, when I was taking on that part of my personality, it was a huge help. I feel like I am going back to where I was as a child, talking a lot and being an impulsive risk-taker, all of which have served me well and have also been a shadow."

Jim, an introvert, talked about the quality in him that challenges Marianne. "I tend to be more thoughtful. One of the things Marianne has endured with me is that I am a procrastinator. Before I do something, I think about it for a long time. But I don't always externalize my thoughts. I keep so much within myself that it can be detrimental to my health. I was raised by a father who was hard and who said, 'If you don't want your feelings hurt, put them in your pocket.' Don't let people know your real feelings. Hide them. If you don't know what I think, you can't criticize me. I don't do it as much as I used to. I am both an introvert and an extrovert. I like people but like alone time, more at night, when the house is quiet—a different kind of quiet. I can have the TV on and don't even know it. I am thinking about what I don't think about during the day. She may understand me spending the nights alone in the basement, but it is still difficult for her. I wish I were more the other way, but I also find I do a lot of talking during the day to different groups. I don't want to burden other people with my problems. Over the years, people asked, 'Why not talk about it?' I can talk, but usually to groups of people, not so much one-on-one."

Being raised in large families, both name the gifts they have in common and their values for living and loving in a community. The values—engendered from childhoods that were filled with many siblings and cousins—include hard work, kindness, loyalty, humor, respect for others' needs, the sense that family has each other's backs, and caring for the less fortunate. They believe that how you treat others is a reflection of your character. Marianne added, "Another core value is being one of many, or as I describe that experience, as one of benign neglect. My parents couldn't focus on just me. That gave me a sense of self as an individual with the freedom to develop my gifts. Consciously and subconsciously, I instilled this in our children as well. You, we, and I have individual gifts. The gift of the gifts is that we take them and develop them for the world. Outward thinking towards the world is at the core of our values." In their 70s and 80s, they now are guided by these values in their service to and presence with others.

Jim and Marianne are deeply committed, not only to each other but to the welfare of others in their community. Jim concluded the reflection on values. "Respecting others is informed by the spiritual value of, 'Do unto others as they do unto you.' That is a value we try to maintain in and outside of family and explains why we have been active in the larger community in different ways. We know we are part of the greater family of our community. Being raised by strict Baptists, I am held to the line. As we have grown older and the world has changed, these values help us cope; they help us continue to exist. But of all the gifts we possess, the most important is kindness and love."

You may be wondering how they are putting these values into action now. Marianne publishes books of her own poetry, leads retreat series for teachers, and mentors for the Center for Courage & Renewal. They are both active in their church and are a part of various support groups. Marianne recounted a story that captures this "elder, beneficial presence" and how she operates as a natural mentor. "I love going shopping at the grocery or dollar stores, but not for clothes. I don't try on clothes. I love the conversations with the young people who work in those places, asking them questions, supporting them, and telling them, 'I think a lot about your world. I don't use plastic.' I talk to them about their education and ask, 'Are you in school? What are you studying?' They love to talk to us oldsters. They love it when we show an interest in them. I said to the young woman who works at the gas station, 'You are looking sleepy today.' And she responds, 'This is my second of three jobs, and I have a baby. I am tired a lot.' It is such a privilege to listen to what she has to say. The learning is immense.

"This is true with older friends too. We have time to listen and learn. We had Howard, age ninety-two, and his partner, eighty-six, for dinner, and we sat at the table for a long time. They were asking Jim questions. He was sharing about his life as an African American male, and we learned together that Sunday evening. Howard could hardly get up but was engrossed in the conversation. We are learning and unlearning what we thought we knew."

Jim still works a few days a month as a substitute teacher in a local high school and, drawing on his background and PhD in accounting, business administration, and public administration, serves on a board of a financial institution he founded with friends. Jim explained that the Community Promise Federal Credit Union is located in the "financial desert" to serve communities of color and immigrants. They make small loans to low-income people needing help starting new businesses, and break the power of payday lenders in the lives of the poor. Jim also initiated a group for minority youths in high school to create a safe space for them to discuss their struggles with school and their minority status, and to prepare for their futures beyond high school.

In his words, "Contact with the younger people is learning in itself. Being in a high school several days a month, you get a new perspective, their perspective, on many things, and it makes you think. Young people today are no different, but they have different toys. I was born in a time when we had no electricity or running water in the house, and no TV either. These young people have all of that, plus more. Their perspective is different, and I learn how they adjust to the world they find. We talk about the world that they live in as people of color, and what they need to do to be successful in this world. I tell them, 'What you do now determines what you will do in the future. The best way to approach life is to prepare yourselves as best you can, in the now.'

"We talk about the unfairness and that no one ever promised you things would be fair. They can expect an unfair world, not just for people of color. Others experience this too. Whatever is out there, how you prepare yourself now will determine how you will cope. Get good grades, and help one another. You may be strong in some subjects, so help others with your strengths and vice-versa. Don't be afraid to ask for help. Sometimes we get white kids, and I have a message for them as well. The world they are entering will be more diverse. Don't be afraid to embrace diversity. It will make you stronger. I enjoy the diversity. It is the world they will be living in. It is a good thing. Even though I teach in an above-average school district, there are still some single-parent families and more economic diversity. In the late '50s, there was no diversity."

While they both are "servant leaders" with hearts of gold, with aging, they find it necessary to turn their service work toward home. Marianne recently suffered from a stroke, and in her mid-80s, she faces many physical challenges. "I think we have arrived at a time in our marriage that love has a big component of service to each other as we age. Because I am ahead of Jim in that department, being older by eleven years,

I wonder what I would do without him. Without each other, where would we be? Love is more than the original emotion, but that is still there. I look into his eyes, or when he is holding a grandchild, I love him more. That is still there, but the need for one another is a good part of love at this time. For instance, he makes the stairs easier than I do. He can carry the laundry up and down them. Ordinary, everyday things, like when Jim gives me his arm when we walk. He offers his accounting ability for my retreat work since the world of finance is not within my bandwidth. I love him for the ways he stepped up after my stroke, with a weakening of my executive powers."

Jim added, "The service is manifested in the little things. 'Do you need a refill on your coffee, or get whatever? I am going to the store.' Realizing Marianne has had a hard day and is tired, I am asking about what I can do. It is about the little things we do to make each other's life more comfortable. Trying to anticipate the needs of the other, and trying to serve each other, becomes more important as we grow older and lose a step or two. So we serve each other."

Vulnerability is essential to authentic intimacy. Jim and Marianne share tender vulnerability at this stage of life, where health and functioning challenges increase. "For better or for worse" is a paradox at the center of aging and relationships—sometimes the "worse" becomes the better times for our souls and in our love for one another.

Addressing our curiosity about their spiritual journeys, Jim and Marianne recalled two stories that explain a great deal of how they encountered the Divine.

Marianne went first. "As a third-grader, when I was about eight, I was a swimmer, and in our small town, the public pool offered free swimming lessons to kids like me in the morning, for we didn't have much money. I never missed a day. My life was the water. Water has always been my element. My mother described me as a baby loving the bath. I loved how it made me feel. One day in June, it was too cold, and my mother said I shouldn't go to my lesson. But I went and was the only child that showed up. The young lifeguard came out wrapped in a towel in sweatpants, then stood by the pool and watched me swim. I remember being in that big pool alone, swimming and cavorting and loving it. Floating on my back, I thought, *This must be how God is holding us.* I've come to think of my experience as unifying for me."

Many spiritually devoted people have childhood stories of their first encounters with the Divine that contain a numinous quality and serve as unforgettable touchstones, easily accessed when recalled. Even though she was eight at the time, Marianne told this story as if it had happened yesterday. Mystical experiences often exist outside of time.

Jim's experience occurred when he was a little older, yet it is still as clear and present as ever. "During my first year in college, I had been finishing school in Kalamazoo, going back to my parents for the weekends, for they lived about 45 miles southwest from here. I was at a party one night. It was two in the morning, and I was driving my old Renault when the bearings went out on my car, a wheel broke off, and the car suddenly dipped down, flipped over, and slid sidewise; I ended up gripping the gearshift. I remember saying out loud, 'Lord, I am coming home.' I was calm as could be. I was not afraid. Once the car stopped, I crawled out through the windshield, and stood by the car, still calm, but when I looked at the car, I started shaking. The car was a mess, but I had not a scratch on me. This was a mystical, miraculous experience.

"I said to myself, 'It isn't my time. Maybe God has other things I am meant to do.' When I look back, the same thought comes to me. It is an experience that has impacted my thinking even about death. Death has given me a second chance, and I am peaceful about death." When you consider how many people are motivated by a fear of death, this is truly a profound, mystical gift Jim received at an early age.

As we continued to investigate spiritual themes, we asked Marianne about her passage from living in a convent as a Sister of Loretto to the present. The story of her spiritual evolution poured out as a far-flung exploration similar to what many baby boomers have undergone. "I was raised in a devout Roman Catholic family, and it served me well, educationally and spiritually. We learned early on not to question doctrine, which served me pretty well with strong boundaries. When I turned eighteen, after twelve years of Catholic education, I decided to become a sister. In my college years, I spent time with and learned from women who were strong, educated, liberal, and more and more progressive; I loved it, and I loved my life. I was so fortunate to have that group of women as mentors. What happened over those thirteen years was a chance to delve deeply into philosophy, history, and church history; there were no boundaries. I freely moved beyond doctrine, and my spirituality developed over that time and in the years that followed.

"With a foundation as an extremely devout Roman Catholic and an education that took the form of broadening and deepening, I was also fortunate to study abroad. I had wonderful professors recognized internationally in their fields. What was happening was the development of my spirituality and my vision of body, mind, soul, and brain functioning. I find myself today saying honestly, 'I am Buddhist, a Hindu, Quaker, Sufi, Jewish, Muslim, and Catholic, not in communion with Rome.' That is where I stand in terms of my spirituality. I don't know if any of those traditions align with where I am spiritually but they all have some input. I could broaden that to other traditions as well."

Like Marianne, many of us elder North Americans began in Protestant, Jewish, or Catholic traditions, which provided helpful boundaries of doctrine and rules, mentors, a sense of belonging, and instructions on how to be, think, live, pray, and what not to do (mostly not to have sex outside of marriage). These things served us well in our youth. Like Marianne, adolescence and the college years led us far afield from these boundaries to new freedom to explore other traditions, which opened up to the West just as we came of age. Eventually, the Dalai Lama reminded us to claim the roots of our traditions, for the sampling of many things would never take us deep enough. Spiritual depth requires a commitment to a path. Jim and Marianne have managed to balance this radical inclusion and openness with a life of devotion within a progressive Catholic congregation.

As our interview came to an end, we were touched by the richness of their lives and their challenges. Looking back at our parents and grandparents, we wonder how they handled this time of life, searching for positive models and clues. Jim told a story about his Grandpa Sang, whom he remembers seeing behind a plow and a mule. He lived to age 103 and was still actively participating in life to his fullest capacity, even at the end.

"I thought about all he had seen, and I knew him as an old man, at 100 years, who was still preaching as a minister. I heard people thought he was dead at 101, but when I visited him in the hospital, he was sitting up smoking a cigar. What was he thinking? When I asked, 'How are you doing, Grandpa?' he remarked, 'I could preach the horns off a billy goat!' There was a spirit there. He recognized the voices of people, even though he was partially blind. He knew the name he had given to each of us. That is why you want to stay vigorous and active."

While Jim and Marianne may not smoke cigars at the end of their days, we are confident they will do everything within their power to share their care, opinions, stories, laughter, questions, and love of life until they pass from this world.

*Try to keep your soul young and quivering right
up to old age, and to imagine right up
To the brink of death that life is only beginning.*

GEORGE SAND

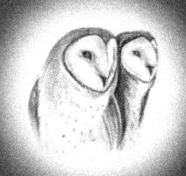

Blessed is the couple who
embraces all seasons of life
—the perennial cycles of spring,
summer, autumn, and winter—
for they shall know wholeness.

BLESSED IS THE COUPLE WHO
Embraces All Seasons of Life

INTRODUCING
CARYL & JEFF CRESWELL

WHEN WE INVITED Caryl and Jeff to be a part of *Side by Side*, Jay and I never envisioned a ribald conversation about sex in old age over a scrumptious dinner. At a bustling Spanish tapas restaurant called Urdaneta that was within walking distance from their home in the Alberta Arts District in Portland, Oregon, we relished a memorable meal. Owned and managed by their daughter, Jael, and son-in-law, Chef Javier, this vibrant, crowded restaurant draws inspiration for the recipes from Javier's native Basque country and love of the rustic tapas bars in the heart of Madrid. Jael greeted us with warm hugs, while Javier indulged us with wave after wave of platters filled with exotic, spicy flavors foreign to our palates, like grilled artichokes seeped in *mojo picon* and sherry aioli. The conversation was even saucier. It must have been the freeing atmosphere, but mid-way through the meal, we lowered our voices to discuss the challenges of sexuality and our older bodies.

We regret that the camera was not rolling but recalled some of the highlights the next day. Caryl noted, "Our discussion last night about sex and aging . . . we are uncomfortable talking about that, but it is a big part of getting older. It was refreshing to sit around in the restaurant and discuss the details, like the awkwardness created by arthritis and our weakened muscles."

Jeff added, "Humorous and true . . . a whole layer of complexity comes with aging and sexuality. You don't move as well as you used to. You need medicinal assistance for this and that. I have never laughed so much as I have with sex at this age. It is not to be seen as embarrassing or as diminishment, but part of the normal changes."

Many assume that at a certain age, couples stop having sex, probably because our generation seldom talks about it. We didn't find this to be the case with our interviewees, and these two were especially forthcoming about the realities. Staying connected sexually and being playful with the challenges enhances intimacy, for it necessitates sharing our vulnerabilities. No one can power through or ignore the physical challenges to our sexuality as we age.

In retrospect, this dinner stands as a metaphor for Caryl and Jeff's relationship and their presence, a feast of family ties with their eight children and grandchildren's lives, infused with their love of fresh food and creative, healthy, homegrown cooking supplied by their backyard garden. Flavored by their international travels and contributions to the world, they share delicious, rich conversations that feed the soul. They are not afraid to go into risky territory of truth-telling, stories, and exploration of many dimensions of living a whole life.

While Caryl and Jeff lived long, full lives before meeting, they share so much in common that they might have been consulting each other along the way. Both dedicated much of their professional lives to the spiritual formation of children, each of them facilitating international programs: Godly Play for Caryl and Storyline International for Jeff. Between the two of them, they raised eight children, endured the deaths of their partners, and practiced active, devoted spiritual lives. As Jeff said, "Something, a force bigger than us, brought us together and nurtures us."

Caryl commented on their beginnings. "I'd been seeing a spiritual director and discussed being lonely, and that I would like to find a life partner. I believe that life is difficult, and we aren't meant to be alone. The spiritual director asked me, 'Are you aware of life circumstances where this might be in front of your eyes, and you aren't aware of it?' So, when I was meeting with Jeff to discuss being a part of a Circle of Trust program, we sat right here in his home and had an amazing conversation. We discovered so many intersections in our lives: we were both widowed, had lots of children, and had similar religious experiences. It was unlike me, but I wrote him an email. That brought us together."

Jeff continued, "I noticed how quickly we went deep in our first conversation, a communion of spirits of two people who have lost spouses. Three weeks later, the emails turned out to be one a day. It went so quickly that after three to four weeks, I planned to visit family in Colorado and asked, 'Would you like to come and meet my family?' She said yes, and within six weeks, we knew we wanted to marry."

In terms of what keeps them together, in addition to their spiritual bond, many values, and a similar sense of vocation, they named the value of commitment in marriage. Caryl said, "We took vows in front of a community to stick it out. Every relationship has struggles. The commitment is critical."

Jeff added, "The commitment is a reliable container for the discord and challenges a couple will face. It's hard to have a long-term relationship without the commitment."

They regret that this current generation of young adults doesn't share this sensibility and express concern about the consequences. They speak from experience, having lived in and through previous challenging marriages. They understand the territory.

Caryl and Jeff must have enviable frequent flyer mileage credits, for every time we reach out to them, we receive texts back from countries like Cuba, Iceland, Scotland, Slovenia, or Mexico. They both uniquely offer to the world their gifts for building community to support children and adults in their spiritual formation. Caryl grew up in Mexico, speaks Spanish, and is a recorded Quaker minister. She pastored Quaker meetings for thirteen years, then worked for twenty years, nationally and internationally, as a trainer for the Godly Play organization, a Montessori-based spiritual education program for children. Jeff and Caryl also lead soul work together through the Center for Courage & Renewal as facilitators, an intersection where their work lives join. Jeff taught elementary school for thirty-two years in Portland and offered training for teachers in the Scottish Storyline curriculum approach. He eventually became the director of this international movement. While many people slow down when they retire from their organizational lives, these two have not.

When we asked how they discern what is important to them now, Caryl began, "I value the question about time and purpose, about what we have energy for and what we do not. We are at the height of our capacity. It is time-limited, and we want to serve intentionally. We want to share our expertise about the importance of children's spirituality. That is where I come alive, and it feeds me and others. It has edges to it because of my far-right Christian upbringing. I do not want to support that old version but become a voice that helps people see Jesus and the Bible in new ways.

When I look back, so much has happened in my life that has brought me to this. I see how the way opens (a Quaker saying) as the support and invitations come to me, which verifies what I am meant to do. We build space and hold space for people to pay attention to their knowing of the Divine and themselves as it reveals itself. There are so few places available for people to do this." It's worth noting that all three of these programs—Storyline, Godly Play, and Circle of Trust—are based on soulful uses of story, literature, art, and writing.

She continued, "We each claim a deep and fundamental belief in the power of story to heal and to enlighten; story is how we learn. While it is fundamental to me, it isn't appreciated or understood in our dominant culture. As Frederick Buechner said, 'My story is important not because it is mine, God knows, but because if I tell it anything like right, the chances are you will recognize that in many ways it is also yours.' I spent two-thirds of my years honing my life, developing my capacity to work with children, and creating safe spaces for adults. I want to pay attention to how to give it away lavishly. I love how we work together. I feel I am growing in my understanding of how, as a couple, we can offer retreats in unique ways that others can't offer. It is very rare for people to experience a couple who can design safe spaces and work together."

In terms of their story as a couple, two years into their relationship, Caryl was diagnosed with Parkinson's disease, which serves as a daily reminder for them about how precious and limited this lifetime is, creating a charged atmosphere for mindfulness about their choices.

As age impacts and impairs the functioning of our bodies, even when we still have a great deal of passion for our interests, illnesses change not only how much work we can do in the world but how we work together as a couple. Many of the interviewees discussed the effect of health problems on their relationships and roles. Caryl and Jeff were especially articulate about the nuances involved when caretaking for one another. Caryl disclosed, "My diagnosis with Parkinson's greatly impacted us. It's not a whole lot different than any other piece of aging. The future will include loss and diminishment. How do you live without being overwhelmed with it, not making it too much of a focus, while addressing what you need to address? I am responsible for making provisions for my condition. It's a tricky balance, not living too much in the future. My biggest anxiety is when I ask, 'What if?' And the need to face, in healthy ways, the fact that we are dying. I have had fear, more of a fear about *how* I will die, not that I will die. I fear the increase of dementia and mental decline with this disease. It is very frightening to me. There are significant memory problems already, like not being able to pull up a name. I get very anxious and wonder if it is a part of Parkinson's or normal aging. Now I am challenged to not grow dark and consumed with anxiety, which destroys the present."

When we asked the couples in our interviews about what they most feared about aging, almost every person said, "Losing my memory." We instinctively intuit how much is lost when our minds go: our personalities, histories, equality in partnerships, and almost all sense of agency and control. Who wouldn't fear this?

Jeff, who spent ten years as a caretaker for his first wife, Sarah, notes, "I am aware of the dance we do. We ask, 'Is this Parkinson's or aging?' I am going through changes too. I will say, 'Me too.' I feel the same way. She has a name for the kind of diminishment she is experiencing. The things happening to her aren't that different from the rest of us. Some have names clumped together as a disease, and the rest of us have normal aging, and they can look much the same. The most important thing is to live in, enjoy, and appreciate the present; live as fully as you are able for as long as you can. Enjoy life out of the fullness you have today. If it changes, you adjust; we will all be adjusting. I have always had an excellent memory. I never kept a calendar for all of the years I taught, for it was in my head. If I don't put it on the calendar now, it's gone. We laugh about how success is only having to go back once rather than twice when leaving the house. My daughter cracks jokes about what I already told her or says things like, 'There goes your memory again.' We wonder if she is a little worried about us. 'It's ok, Dad, you are old.' Who wants to hear that?"

As couples age, we grow subtle antennae for picking up warning signs of slippage and decline in ourselves and each other, silently wondering if that repeated story or failure to recall the name of the movie we just watched reflects encroaching dementia. Our kids grow antennae too. We fear losing each other while we are still alive. We dread becoming a burden. In healthy relationships, we openly discuss these fears, laugh together at our misfires, and extend mercy to this condition called aging.

Caryl noted, "Sometimes I have said, 'I am not Sarah.' Jeff is a caretaker. I want him to be aware but not move into a caretaking mode that diminishes more of who I am. It's an issue with aging. It's not helpful when caretaking becomes over-protection. It feels like it puts you into an inequitable relationship. Recently an aunt of mine suffered from dementia. Her husband took on a role that exacerbated it. How do we respect that person's dignity when caretaking? We should guard and respect each other when there are losses, both mental and physical."

Jeff recalled the ten years of tending to Sarah through her decline with a rare immune disorder. "There is also the fact that when you do commit to caring for each other, you can get to a place where you go into it so much that you lose perspective on what's happening. It's important to know when to ask for help. 'I need a break. I can't do this by myself.' Reflecting on my experience with Sarah, it never occurred to me to ask for help. I didn't know I needed help. When she died, I experienced the grief of losing my wife compounded by the grief of losing my role. Caregiving had become a primary role over parent and teacher. I had lost both my wife and my role as a caregiver; I felt empty. I wondered, 'What do I do now that both are gone?' It was really scary. I think of my parents; Dad is ninety-three, and Mom is ninety-one. Both struggle with admitting they need help, let alone asking for it. My father should be using a cane; he can hardly walk, but he refuses to use one. They installed an electric lift chair to go upstairs; he won't use it. It takes him ten minutes to go up the stairs. When will I get to a place where I shouldn't drive anymore? At times, I am on the edges of that, like at night. When I was driving at night to Kirkridge Retreat Center in Pennsylvania during a horrible storm, I kept going when I should have stopped. I was going to power through this. I shouldn't have done that. I want to figure out how to avoid making that mistake again."

Caryl and Jeff have navigated more than their share of loss, both currently with Caryl's diagnosis and their experiences with losing a spouse. Jeff lost Sarah three years before he met Caryl, while it had been eighteen years since Caryl's husband died by suicide, leaving her to raise their five children alone.

We asked them to comment on what it was like becoming a widow and widower since we are all in the time of life when we will either die first or be left widowed in the future. Many couples discuss how the other will fare without each other and who wants to go first. We wonder about how to be around our widowed friends. Caryl and Jeff shed some light on these oft-private musings.

Caryl began, "When people ask me about being widowed, I share that we have gone through it and are fairly intact human beings. After a loss like this, you need to have a place to speak of things that are going on within you. The second year after the death, for me, was even harder than the first year. That there is a time limit to grief is a false notion. It never gets resolved in some ways. It is a good two years where life is suspended, and your emotions and energy are taken up. Help people with that, if you can. Naming those pieces for them is a gift. Grief is some of the hardest work we do. Permit people to undergo this difficult work."

Jeff continued, "I say to those in grief, 'Whatever you are going through is normal. Your grief is your grief. Be selfish. Take care of yourself. Ignore the things people say.' You don't get over it; you just learn how to carry it better. Even so, it can still knock you off your feet. It will always be that way. People fall away; they stop contacting you because they don't know what to say or do. 'What to say or do' are the wrong questions. The most significant gift you can give someone who is grieving is being in their presence without trying to fix them. The worst thing you can do is to ask them what you can do. It puts it on them. They need food, beauty, and clothing; don't ask them if you can help. Bring them a pot of soup. It will be greatly appreciated. After Sarah's funeral, I remember a long queue of people wanting to see me. I was doing all of the work. At the beginning of my grieving process, I was grieving 24/7. The funeral was me helping other people. Grief and a loss are not something to get over nor a problem to fix."

Caryl concluded with this final insight. "One thing is from my religious background. I was so offended when people took a religious concept and fed it to me. 'God must have known how strong you are to give you this trial.' Causality?

God, the puppeteer? Really? Avoid religious platitudes. They are really offensive."

While none of us want to consider losing our partners, most of us quietly ruminate about it. It offers a reminder to enjoy each other while we can. Jeff was transparent about how challenging it was to be left alone after many years of marriage and family life. "The biggest hole in my life after losing my first wife was being alone. Every day I felt a crushing aloneness. I had to initiate and make choices all of the time to be with other people. It was exhausting. Having that other person there in the everydayness is a huge gift. Because that kind of love is so nourishing and generative, it allows you to reach out to others because we have this well to draw from at home."

We are so grateful for their honesty and transparency of these realities of aging and loss.

In our work through the Center for Courage & Renewal, we often talk about the notion of reconnecting soul and role, interweaving what we love and our sense of calling to what we do. For Caryl and Jeff, their professional lives intermingle with their spiritual practices. For example, in Godly Play, they rely on what they name "wondering questions" when telling a Bible story to aid children in discovering its meaning. Caryl and Jeff use wondering questions from Godly Play to touch in with themselves and each other at the end of each day.[1]

The Four Wondering Questions
What was the best part of the day?
What was the most important part of the day?
What was just for you?
What could you have left out?

Caryl added that in addition to reflecting on these questions, "We read a spiritual book out loud together at night, like one of Brian Doyle's collections of essays. It is amazing to have Jeff to talk and wrestle with when we are exposed to new ideas."

Jeff noted that, "We are always processing our work and family life on a spiritual level, asking ourselves, 'How are we growing? What are our edges?' To go through experiences together and examine how we are changing, all are an important part of how we are with each other."

Yet, while they both claim Christianity as their faith tradition, they worship and engage their practices separately, and at times quite differently. They both struggle with their early upbringing and religious indoctrinations and have, over time, charted their individual paths to stay connected with Spirit. In Caryl's words, "The deconstruction of Christianity and God is an ongoing piece of our journey, including breaking out of a limited, conservative theology to a more open approach [which] is important to us."

Jeff built on this line of thought: "And loving the pieces of our past we do share. It is beautiful to have this common background. Marianne Borg has a saying, 'I am a Jesus girl, who called me early.' We are Jesus people too, but we have let go of much of what we were taught. Caryl says that Godly Play is her spiritual practice. I want to affirm that. It's not just when she is in a circle telling stories, but the fact that our whole garage and basement are full of things for Godly Play. She is creating stories to tell to others. It's not just paint and glue. She is constantly reflecting on how she needs to support others in communities where they need help recognizing the innate, deep spirituality that is in all children (and everyone) through story.

"For myself, there has been a whole evolution of practices beginning with daily devotions. In my tradition, there were specific ways you were to pray, and to read the Bible; I dutifully did that, but it wasn't working, so I threw out everything.

You have to pay attention to what your heart calls you to and see what happens. I started journaling thirty years ago. It fed me, but I became hungry for more. I took a class at Trinity Episcopal Cathedral in Portland with Marianne Borg on Centering Prayer. I went to that class for five years before I thought I could sit independently. I could sit in groups but was too hyper to sit alone. My contemplative practice grew from that. Now I sit thirty minutes in the morning and twenty minutes in the evening. I also use a series of set prayers. I knew I wanted prayer time but was bounded by the 'create your own prayer' thing. It didn't work for me. I found written prayer and use a Celtic daily prayer book. I use prayers from Iona, Scotland, readings in the Psalms and Gospels, and then I journal. This evolved over time, to let go of expectations of what it ought to be."

"Part of my history entails a regular visit to a Trappist monastery," Caryl said. "A year after my husband's death by suicide, when my father was dying from cancer, my sister visited with her four kids, which made nine children in the house. It was an incredibly intense time. A friend called and offered me a chance to stay at the Trappist Monastery in Carlton, Oregon. She had a reservation and couldn't go, so I went. It was this incredible homecoming, something about sitting in silence with the monks. I heard many words that were so hurtful after Kevin's death. It was very restorative to just be in this silence, in this monastery. I then went monthly for twenty years, and it saved my life. When I got tired and grouchy, my kids would ask, 'Isn't it time to go to the monastery?' I want to reestablish that in my life."

Jeff and Caryl currently each see a spiritual director. "My faith community is at West Hills Quaker meeting of Portland," said Caryl, "a bunch of quirky Quakers doing work that matters in the world. They have recorded me, noticed my gifts, named, valued, and spoken of them." Jeff worships at Trinity Episcopal Cathedral.

Many Christian faith traditions have focused more on beliefs than practices, on "faith" rather than experience, but this is beginning to change with movements like Centering Prayer, pilgrimages, and Lectio Divina, a prescribed, personal approach to reading scripture. Christianity is starting to reclaim some of its mystical, contemplative roots and practices. Service to others, and the connection of soul and role, are organically woven into both Caryl and Jeff's lives and are inspirited by their contemplative practices.

They humorously noted that while they have both changed and grown out of their evangelical Christian roots, they still enjoy spending a whole evening singing "bad evangelical songs." Jeff and Caryl struggled mightily with the deformation of Christianity, yet hold their relationship with God as central to their bond, as a container for their relationship.

Jeff reflected, "When thinking about the possibility of finding a partner, I knew that this would be the deal-breaker for me. It wasn't going to work without a foundational relationship with the Divine."

Caryl concluded, "It's a core piece of our individuality and relationship."

Caryl and Jeff embody so many qualities, values, and practices that healthy couples embrace: self-honesty, commitment, offering goodness and beneficial presence to the world, loving their family and friends, supporting and respecting each other along the way, and a deep, active devotion to Spirit.

As we concluded their interview, Jeff summed up his thoughts about what has built a foundation of trust in a later-in-life marriage. "I think we have done some significant, challenging work together, like crafting a will with a blended family, combining two households, and wrestling with our different attitudes towards money. I don't think we do a good job of acknowledging how well we have done. It is messy and hard, but we have done it well. The ability to love one another's children is key. I love my children's relationship with Caryl and am overwhelmed by the beauty of how Caryl is building a connection with them. The first time we visited Joel, Sibly, and baby Sophie, only two weeks old, Caryl asked, 'What would you like Sophie to call me?' Joel said, 'Grandma Nana.' The fact that he wants her to be a grandmother, now that's pretty sweet."

*Questions are lanterns we swing
ahead of us to see in the dark.*

MARK NEPO

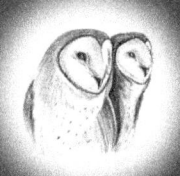

Blessed is the couple who
welcomes the stranger in
each other, for they shall find
wonder and encouragement
on their growing edges.

BLESSED IS THE COUPLE WHO
Welcomes the Stranger

INTRODUCING
LAURIE RUTENBERG & GARY SCHOENBERG

WHEN WE INVITED Laurie and Gary out on a "date" to mutually discern if they would be willing to be interviewed for *Side by Side*, they insisted on hosting us for lunch in their home. Pulling up to *Gesher* (the Hebrew word for "bridge"), their house in the hills of Portland, Oregon, we found them working in the kitchen, preparing an elaborate, homemade meal for us. Before sitting down, we stood at a table with candleholders, and they explained to us that they had gathered around these candles as Shabbat began the evening before.

Even though it was Shabbat day, they invited us to stand before these candleholders and name something we were grateful for. When we mentioned that our daughter was pregnant with her first child, they shouted, 'Mazel tov!' and warmly hugged us. We chanted prayers and sang a song while Gary played the guitar, then ritually washed our hands and were treated to a loaf of challah, delicious savory soups, and salads, one course at a time over three hours.

At the time, we didn't know exactly what was going on, but we recognized a blessing when we saw one. This was no regular lunch but a rare, radical gift of hospitality. By the end of the meal, we crossed over the gesher and moved from being strangers to friends, toasting with their sweet homemade wine our decision to go ahead with the interview.[1]

Soon, we realized this lunch was a microcosm of their life's work, which they claim as "welcoming the stranger." It stands as a metaphor for how they live as a couple, both on the outside and within. Recognizing the act of sharing a meal as an ancient, fundamental custom for building and restoring good relationships, Gary and Laurie have hosted Shabbat meals and other Jewish celebrations and rituals for over 8,500 unaffiliated or intermarried Jews, modeling and passing on their traditions in this home-grown fashion. We felt deeply honored to be invited to this table.

A "locution" is a word that creates an experience of what it means. "Welcome" is one of those words, for just saying it opens a space between people. Gary and Laurie practice and embody "welcome." It is who they are.

When we asked them to share their story of coming together, they noted that they were young strangers when they met in rabbinical school in Jerusalem, and they didn't like each other much, at first. Gary was living in a dorm for observant Jews but confessed that he wasn't exactly observant at the time. Laurie was looking for other students who took Jewish learning seriously—she had aspired to the rabbinate since before women were admitted—and was shocked when Gary didn't know of the Mishnah (the Jewish text that forms the basis for the development of post-Biblical Judaism). She viewed him with disappointment and judgment, privately asking a friend how he had gotten into this school. For six years, their time in school occupied them, and their relationship didn't grow. However, in the last half of the final year, their dormant relationship began to blossom. Nonetheless, upon graduation, Laurie and Gary went their own ways to begin their careers.

Following ordination/graduation, Laurie became the assistant chaplain at Yale University, the first non-Protestant clergyperson, and the first rabbi to ever serve in that role. Gary worked as a rabbi of a small synagogue in Livermore, California. Despite the distance, their bond grew, assisted by many coast-to-coast visits. One year later, they married in Florida, where Laurie's family resided, on July 4, 1982, which Gary dubbed "interdependence day."

Couples with two highly skilled professionals in the same field are presented with challenges when it comes to finding work in the same community. Gary offered to make the first career compromise in their relationship and left the rabbinic position in Livermore, which he loved, to join Laurie and support her in continuing her position at Yale, where she was promoted to Associate University Chaplain. Gary then worked as a rabbinic fellow at the National Jewish Center for Learning and Leadership (Clal), commuting to New York City. Three years later, it was time for Laurie to make a career compromise. Gary wanted to be near his family in Los Angeles, so they moved, and he became the associate rabbi at a large urban congregation in Hollywood, while she served as the Hillel director for Cal State Northridge. Finally, in 1990, they moved to Portland, Oregon, to establish Gesher, where they raised their two children, Avital Shira and Michael Lev.

The rabbis had many bridges to cross in their relationship, just as all couples do, and sometimes encountered each other as strangers, both in background and temperament. A story about registering for chinaware when they were about to be married captures the contrast in how they were reared.

Laurie's childhood family only ate together once a week for their Shabbat dinner due to her father's business demands, but on these occasions, they always ate on fine porcelain plates at an elegantly set table, with different dishes for each course. In sharp contrast, Gary's family dined together every night, buffet style. The dishes wandered to the table—if they were the same, it was a random event, and they scarfed down their food in twenty minutes. Gary grew up surrounded by chaos, influenced by a manic-depressive, alcoholic father and the trauma of his five-year-old brother's death after being hit by a car.

When Laurie's mother suggested they register for plates before the wedding, Gary, a child of the '60s, wondered, "Who am I marrying, Nancy Reagan?" Chinaware symbolized something dramatically different to each of them. In the end, Gary came to understand that he and Laurie had very different relationships with the same symbol (a plate of china). For him, it represented formal and unrelaxed situations. Holidays, which were the few times in a year when his mother brought out the china, were the times his family was most stilted and strained. For Laurie, eating on china was the time of deepest connections. Understanding this, he decided that he'd be open to registering for china, but Laurie never fully trusted his "conversion," so they didn't register. It was not a total surprise to them, after their wedding, that they received four different sets of dinnerware, all from Laurie's side of the family, which to this day, they use to serve their community Shabbat meals.

Gary realized that the pandemonium of his family's ways created a sense of loneliness for him, and a longing for meals where people would truly connect. He discovered a powerful model of creating connections on Shabbat and holidays in the dorms in Jerusalem and in the family homes of observant Jews he met there. Laurie was inspired by the Shabbat meals at the homes of some of her professors' families in college, which added greatly to her vision of what she hoped to create in her future family life. Over time, Gary came to appreciate the nuances and value of a beautifully adorned table and the way a meal is served. They have both come to realize the strengths as well as the deficits of their family upbringings. At the core of their relationship and village life at Gesher is a fusion of the wisdom from both of their backgrounds and lives, and their differing gifts and longings.

In Laurie's presence, her soft-spoken, reflective, quiet nature exudes depth, warmth, and kind, respectful attentiveness. Gary radiates enthusiasm and charisma, and is brightly articulate, gregarious, and adventurous. They are both wickedly intelligent. When we asked them to name an animal that captures the spirit of their partner, Gary designated Laurie as "An owl and eagle. They are predators, wisdom in flight. Laurie has owl wisdom in her, and the elegant flight of an eagle."

For Gary, Laurie said, "Squirrels chasing each other around fir tree trunks. Gary is so playful. Or a growling bear, and sometimes when he wants his own time to be contemplative, a cat. Gary is a chimpanzee, wise in a social way."

Couples are infamously attracted to their opposites, providing a rich ground for learning that often entails conflict and negotiation. Our differences stretch us. If we learn to take advantage of them, and see them as teachers, they enrich our lives. Gary summarized, "She brings a centeredness and heart connection that builds community. I bring passion, music, a sense of humor, and an ability to focus on a question." One of Gary's favorite sayings is, "Every question is a quest."

A couple's differences are the hard ground they walk on, with the "questing" questions about how to honor and benefit from their contrasting worldviews, gifts, and temperaments.

As we age, these differences don't go away, but in fact become more apparent. If we fail to work respectfully with differences, we can become strangers to each other.

One time when staying at Breitenbush Hot Springs, a retreat center in an old-growth forest in Oregon, Laurie decided to join Gary in one of his favorite activities: mushroom hunting. They headed out late one afternoon, and she didn't pack up the normal things she usually would for a hike, since Gary assured her they would only be out for a half-hour. Absorbed in the grandeur of the ancient fir trees, she noticed the sun was setting quickly, and that it was time to get back. Disoriented in the darkening, dripping rainforest, they took a wrong turn and lost their way, forcing them to spend that autumn night under a downed tree in the woods. Gary tried to keep Laurie awake to fight off hypothermia, while she slept on top of him to keep them warm; she awoke with snow on her back.

For Laurie, it was one of the most stressful nights she has endured, but she also noted that they enjoyed meaningful conversations and felt more bonded in the end. For Gary, it was an adventure. He reports that he has been lost many times mushroom hunting, and he never felt their lives were threatened. Couples often have different stories about the same events. We found that Gary and Laurie allowed each other to tell their stories differently while standing their ground.

It is as though each person in a couple poises on opposite sides of a footbridge—how they cross that bridge makes the difference between moving closer or farther away, towards becoming strangers. Laurie takes a step that is essential to moving closer, both to Gary, and herself. While angry and frustrated, ultimately, instead of blaming Gary for getting lost, she looked at how her choices influenced the outcome. Her intuition told her to pack up water, food, and warm clothing, as she always does, before taking a hike. She over-rode that intuition. In her words, "This was a risk I took with Gary, trusting it would be a thirty-minute walk. I let myself be convinced it would be safe. I didn't stick to my guts and wasn't prepared." With compunction and humility, she reflects on other times she has not listened to her inner guidance, with equally unsatisfying results. She engaged in what we call shadow work. Had she blamed Gary, the distance between them would have been more difficult to bridge.

Laurie commented, "We have to be strangers sometimes for us to come together. We can get very out of sync, start not seeing life from a shared perspective, and on the surface, at least, become focused on a disagreement. When this happens, dissonance develops between us as we attend to what we are doing individually, but we start to miss each other. We can be in the same house and not see each other because we have each started to close down."

Laurie names another often unspoken but obvious truth about long-term, committed relationships: we change. "A stranger is someone new. The wonderful thing about welcoming the stranger is that we see something new in each other and welcome the newness, the growth. I am not who I was two minutes ago, and I can be open to the growth of whom we are both becoming. We need to know how to welcome what is new in us, and it's important we share it. When Gary does this for me, it is a gift that makes me feel grateful." In strong relationships, couples encourage one another in what they are becoming, on their growing edges, even if it is threatening or disturbing. This is especially important with the changes that are inherent in growing older.

Laurie and Gary's relationship entwined their work lives when they created Gesher in their home, literally going public as a couple in ways that remain private for most of us. They generously shared their home, family life, rich Judaic traditions, and their leadership. While they started with separate careers as rabbis, when they manifested Gesher, they faced the power dynamics and tensions that workplaces present. Bridging their differences in terms of aptitudes, perceptions, expectations regarding gender roles, and differing gifts was yet another opportunity for them to negotiate change over time. The baby boomer generation forged new ground in gender roles and professional identities, which today are easy to forget.

Laurie's and Gary's differentiated roles helped Gesher flourish but also led to what felt in some ways like an imbalance of influence, even though over time they learned from each other and their roles became more fluid. The rabbis openly discuss the power imbalance that developed as a result of some of their early decisions and divergent gifts. Now, they gratefully celebrate and honor each other's strengths, growth, and contributions to the whole. Their understanding of their rabbinate includes an ongoing address of these imbalances and the recognition that the hard work to support each other in doing so benefits all.

Gesher follows the John Dewey model of education, teaching through experience and example. Their curriculum is a mixture of reclamation and reformation of their traditions, and their mission is to help other Jews practice their Jewish life in ways that work today. For the generation raised in the '50s and '60s, many attended synagogue or church each weekend with their parents and ate regular meals their mothers prepared for the family. We find it hard to comprehend how now, sitting down together for a home-cooked meal is a disappearing norm. Or that observing the ancient customs of the Sabbath by abstaining from work to attend to our loved ones and our relationship with God would become countercultural. Yet in this world of 24/7 internet connectivity, mass exodus from our religious centers, and an out-of-balance work ethic that consumes our lives, the practices of breaking bread together, slowing down, or staying home to observe the Sabbath are radical moves. At least one in five Jews claim no religious affiliation. At Gesher, Gary and Laurie invite people home to the essence of their tradition, and model ways to practice that are rich, relevant, and needed today.

As we looked forward to interviewing Gary and Laurie, we wondered if some of their practices might enrich couples reading this book. We weren't disappointed. They taught us about Yom Kippur, a day of atonement that focuses on self-examination and asking for forgiveness. Couples don't thrive without a strong capacity for forgiveness. Laurie and Gary developed a creative approach that sustains their relationship, family life, and spiritual growth as well.

Laurie noted, "Gary has said I am slow to forgive, and there is something to that. I am slow to apologize because it wouldn't be genuine unless I had true clarity about what I was saying I am sorry for. I want to have a clear awareness of what I did that hurt or caused him harm, so I won't repeat it. I feel bad both for what I did and for not even being aware of it. No real repair is possible if we don't know and deeply understand what we are apologizing for."

Gary added, "I encounter couples who are stuck for years due to their inability to deal with the damage they have created for each other. Laurie and I would see a family therapist periodically, like a doctor, to help us with our ability to be forgiving, and seeking forgiveness has grown with us, as a couple."

Laurie continued, "Gary and I have created a practice that helps us as a couple and as a family with the process of forgiveness. It is built upon our understanding of the richness and fruitfulness of the traditional experience of the Jewish holy day of Yom Kippur, also known as the 'Sabbath of Sabbaths,' the holiest day of the year in Judaism. Its central themes are repentance and atonement. It is a day when the entire Jewish community asks for and supports one another in praying for forgiveness for all our wrongs of the previous year, but we do this with an understanding that God will not be forgiving for wrongs if we haven't first made amends with the other person and then asked them for forgiveness.

"In this context, Gary wrote a letter to me early in our marriage in anticipation of Yom Kippur, about the things he regretted and was sorry for. Soon after, we began an annual practice of writing letters to one another, which we call *Teshuvah* letters. Teshuvah means "return" or realignment with what is holy in each of us, but is really about the repair of our soul with the Holy One, realigning with our best selves. We have written these letters every year (addressing the Holy One, and each other).

"This became so deeply beautiful and meaningful that when we had children, we expanded the practice and started to write to our children as well. From the time of their infancy through today (thirty-three years later), we tell them in these letters how we have witnessed both their growth and also their struggles, and how we are proud of them. Our goal is to give them love, guidance, and courage. We also share the actions that we regret, say how we will try to make amends, and ask for forgiveness. We say 'I'm sorry,' and that we love them. We name the ways we have seen growth in each other, too.

"I write these letters out of love, and I feel very loved in receiving them from Gary. Gary or I write the letters at other times during the year as well, if a moment seems to call for them."

That Judaism claims Yom Kippur as its most holy of days acknowledges how central forgiveness is to relationships in order to stay current with each other, so you can "return" to a new place to begin again. So often, when we are angry, in need of forgiveness, or disappointed in ourselves and each other, there is also some inner work calling us to attend to an unresolved issue. Forgiveness becomes another question and quest—rarely a quick fix, but a process that lasts over time, with layer after layer of nuanced meaning. As couples grow older, they look in the rearview mirror for the damage they have left behind in relationships and seek forgiveness and repair, clearing the road ahead for peace within.

Most of us know of the Sabbath but are uninformed about its origins and potential. Gary began, "Judaism's home-based practices of the Sabbath fuel us as a couple, and that is what people experience in our home. We hug our children. That is a revelation for some. We bless our children. That is new for most. When you are swimming upstream culturally, people recognize, 'Oh, I am hungry for that.'" In their home, on the Sabbath, they disconnect from the internet, try to avoid work, and focus on their relationships with each other, their children, their community, nature, and God.

Laurie added, "Parenting has been a shared journey. It has allowed us to experience life's deepest blessings. In almost all ways, we honor each other's parenting."

Gary noted, "We work together, and we complement each other in sharing the goal of identifying our children's passions and helping them hone their gifts. We endeavor to help them understand that every challenge is also a spiritual opportunity. An unexpected consequence of our children helping us welcome so many different strangers into their home is that their core self-esteem is so deep."

Gary concluded, "We have encountered people who are a generation or two away from a family meal that worked. We all know the pain in that reality. Two-career madness, single parent challenges, fast food living (which is fast food dying, really). So how does Judaism's wisdom tradition inform us? Judaism is the wisdom of a nomadic tradition, even though they weren't necessarily nomads, but it embraces the changes in the world as challenges and opportunities. So that is what is exciting. The experience of Shabbat in our home, in any Jewish home, provides us a centering point as we navigate through whatever changes in life we experience."

In these challenging times, perhaps the rabbis are wayfinders for all of us, for returning home to what matters most. They model for us how that which makes life sacred and holy is the quality of love, attention, and devotion we give to ordinary actions. A meal is only food until we make it sacred by suffusing it with prayer, careful preparation, and loving attention, offered in a community. Being Jewish also includes a careful choice of what to eat and not eat, in observance of Jewish practices of keeping kosher. Observing the Sabbath makes time sacred by slowing us down. In reducing the speed, we sit with what is happening in our lives, setting aside action to make room for contemplation.

Laurie disclosed how their capacity for Sabbath, and holding space for their questions, served them through their challenges. "When we experienced infertility, and after the death of yet another of Gary's brothers while he was a surgical resident, we sat in pain with Abraham's question in the Torah: 'How will I know that my future is assured by you, God?' The Torah is replete with questions that don't have immediate answers. The holiness of the question is something I came to know through Gary. I don't always need an answer, especially not a final answer, but rather to keep a question alive in our lives. In our relationship, it matters a lot to me to have the willingness to keep exploring questions that matter to us."

Perhaps no other experience in life needs sacred time more than when we face the death of a parent or loved one. Laurie and Gary reflected on their mothers' deaths, and how they extended their home to Laurie's mother to care for her as she transitioned from this life. Since most of us first enter an apprenticeship with death by witnessing our parents die, we asked our couples to share these stories.

Laurie's mother was originally living in a residential home nearby, but they decided when she was actively dying and needed full-time care to move her in with them. Laurie noted, "The greatest love Gary gave me was welcoming her into our home."

"Life deteriorated for her," Gary continued, "as a woman of immense wisdom and control throughout life. Having her in our home gave our children opportunities to be with her. She proceeded to take herself off all medication, which she needed to stay alive." A few months before, she had told Laurie that she had enjoyed a full life and that she felt ready to go. At death's door, with her sons coming in the next morning, the hospitalist told her about a drug that could keep her alive for twenty-four hours, but she wouldn't feel good initially. She said 'yes,' and by morning, she was back at our home from the hospital and was holding court. She had Shabbos dinner with us, and then, after Shabbat lunch the next day, surrounded by all of us at her bedside, she said, 'It is bye-bye time.' She waved, and didn't wake up the next morning."

Laurie pondered, "I wish I had a recording of all of the things she said. She talked about tickets, packing, going home, and being journey-ready. She looked in the closet and declared that she was giving her fur coat to my brother's wife, saying, 'I want you to have this coat.' This was powerful because my brother and parents had once been estranged. Even though our mother, years before, welcomed him back into her life, with that symbolic gesture at death's door, I felt it was an absolute and unequivocal embrace of my brother. She was very graceful and dignified."

The dying often employ symbolic language to let those around them know they are preparing for the journey into death. Packing bags, preparing to leave, going home, and opening windows are all metaphors for departure. We can listen carefully to people at this stage, and respect these warnings for what they are.

Laurie's mother exited with great dignity, fully conscious of what she was doing, and intentionally tying up unfinished business with her formerly estranged son. It stands as a powerful example of "death with dignity." Many families attempt to hide death, not only from themselves but from their children. Having Laurie's mother at home, their children learned that death is normal and can even be beautiful, offering some of life's most tender moments. We have outsourced so many natural family functions, especially around the end of life, but not Laurie and Gary. Those of us who companioned our parents through this transition also learned how to face our end of life, now in the not-so-distant future.

Each death is unique, and none of us know how we will die. When Gary's mom was widowed, he helped her as she adjusted to her new status. "My mom was a certified pain-in-the-tuchus, often my tuchus. In her eighties after Dad died, I helped her understand her finances, taught her how to drive again after a knee replacement left her feeling disoriented and less confident, and called every day. I asked her about what she did today. She was deathly afraid of being alone. After some time adjusting to widowhood, she came alive, delighting in her own company, driving her car, and [inviting] younger friends to classes, museums, and plays. When she turned ninety, I wrote a preview of her eulogy, including ribald humor. It talked about how she employed the FBI ("the Family Bureau of Investigation") and didn't even need wiretapping; she just looked at you, and you felt guilty. While undergoing an optional surgery, she suffered a massive stroke that destroyed half of her brain, and the doctors advised the family to let her die. A disagreement ensued since she did not leave clear instructions for her end-of-life care."

Many of our couples were adamant about how much they fear becoming a burden to their children, yet in truth, we usually need help in some way at the end of our lives. Laurie and Gary's stories reflect how it is soulful and important to care for parents. As we age, we have to surrender our rugged self-reliance, learn how to receive care, and in the process, allow our deaths to become teachers for our children.

Looking back, Gary reflected, "I have done so many funerals, my mom lovingly called me Rabbi Death. It seemed every time she called, I was officiating at a funeral. But, despite my experience with death and dying, I didn't talk with my mom about what she wanted in the event of not being able to have the same quality of life. We were left with her having signed a medical release form without knowing her feelings and opinions about it. When she had her stroke, it made knowing what to do pretty complicated. She left the decision in my brother's hands because she said I was too religious. When she was hooked up to a feeding tube and couldn't talk, or use the right side of her body, and she couldn't care for herself, these were conditions that weighed on us. To this day, I have mixed feelings about ending her life."

In terms of Jewish customs at the time of death, Laurie said, "The acts that we do for a person who has died are considered the truest kindness of all because the dead can't do anything in return. This has to do with the ways the body is cared for. We kept Mom's body in our home, and people sat by her and said Psalms for twenty-four hours. Then we put her on a plane to Florida. When she arrived, a group of volunteers washed the body in a ritual manner, then dressed her in plainness of garb, and put her in a simple casket. Then we had a funeral. The eulogy is very important. Everyone participates in filling the grave. There is a seven-day mourning period, with meals and praying. At the end of the first seven days of mourning, spent inside one's home with the community coming to give comfort, the mourner takes a symbolic walk around the block, reflecting a readiness to shed some of the intensity of the grieving. Then there are thirty days more of less intense grieving, and then, a whole year of practices through which one is known as a mourner in the community."

In a society that gives employees three days' leave to mourn a death, and pressures us to "get over it" as soon as possible, the Jewish customs for burial and mourning reflect the actual needs of a soul deeply disrupted and disoriented when losing a loved one: spacious time, the embrace of the community, and active lamentation. This time-bounded container offers markers for the different stages of grief. Instead of avoiding death, they literally "handle it" by washing and caring for the body, sitting with the body, and participating in burying the body. As we do all of these things, our souls begin to catch up to the new reality, that this person is no longer in their body, no longer with us physically. They have transitioned to a nonmaterial existence that we cannot see. These rituals honor the stages of grief that stretch out over time.

Two of our interview questions are, "How have you prepared for your death?" and "What kind of conversations have you had about your desires around end-of-life?" We found that most couples had not yet discussed this topic, Gary and Laurie included. They admitted that they have a lot of work to do in this area. They concluded our conversations about death by noting that it is a Jewish tradition to write an ethical will, which names what have been the most important values in one's life. In this will, you leave behind a wish for each person you love for what you hope for them, and the qualities you want to pass along. You say what you might wish to say to them when you are no longer here. It includes what you wish you could have done differently, and what you would like them to have.

To everything, there is a season. As with each visit, it was sad for us to end our time with the rabbis. As we did, they were alive with new plans as they acknowledged that the season for growing and tending Gesher was coming to an end. Soon after, they put their property on the market.

Looking forward, Gary anticipates focusing on his writing, sharing stories he has captured along the way to show how Gesher offered powerful antidotes to the loneliness plaguing so many today, as well as preparing the children's books he has written for publication. He foresees having more fun mushroom hunting, fishing, traveling to the nooks and crannies of other cultures, reading, and spending time with Laurie, their children, and close friends. He is ready to step out of the fray of work-centered life.

Laurie is also interested in writing about the fruits of their efforts, meeting with families who attended Gesher, and discovering its influences and impact. She would like to work more closely with and for women, find more time for friendships, their relationship, and their children. Since they have worked with so many groups of "strangers," she looks forward to more time to go in-depth with a few chosen friends. She wants to play the viola and find a study partner who will share her passion for Jewish spiritual learning.

Jay and I carry a burden of sadness and remorse about the ways many Christian institutions discriminated against and persecuted Jews. In this shameful process, it disregarded and distanced from its deep roots in Judaism, cutting Christians off from so much wisdom and history, and depriving us of practices that we are paying for dearly today. The gift of being with and learning from Gary and Laurie continues to teach us as a couple. We now observe our Sabbath with a Shabbat ritual and dinner every weekend. We are so grateful, and celebrate how they are a blessing to the many strangers they have welcomed at Gesher and in their home and hearts dedicated to God and love.

Welcoming guests is even more important than communing with God.

THE BABYLONIAN TALMUD,
RABB YEHUDAH SAID IN THE NAME OF RAV

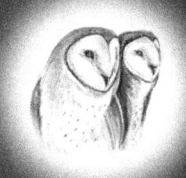

Blessed is the couple who
confronts their own shadows,
for they shall be freed
from blame and projection.

BLESSED IS THE COUPLE WHO

Confronts Their Own Shadows

INTRODUCING
PAUL & ROZ DUMESNIL

DOWN THE BLOCK from where Steve Jobs once lived, in Palo Alto, California, we met Paul and Roz Dumesnil for the first time in the Craftsman home they purchased in 2016. It is a home where they each offer spiritual direction, host grandchildren as well as gatherings small and large, and embrace this time of life with eyes wide open. With most of the couples we interviewed, we have enjoyed some relationship history. In their case, a friend and minister at the nearby Presbyterian Church in Portola Valley, Jenny Warner, told us about Paul and Roz and why she thought they were perfect for this project. She was right. And they dared to show up for us, two camera-toting strangers.

We soon learned how their lives never strayed far from Silicon Valley, for they met nearby fifty-three years ago at Santa Clara University. Two weeks into their first year, they noticed one another and soon became friends. From the start, it was clear how they differed in personality. Roz tended to be more reserved, while Paul was outgoing and gregarious. Paul's buddies liked to "party till you drop." Roz's friends were studious and serious. Yet they found common ground in their spirituality, and as their friendship grew, they began to attend Mass together each afternoon at the Mission on campus. They also discovered a mutual appetite for deep, heart-to-heart conversations. On their first date, they recall seeing the film *The Pawnbroker*, a demanding, evocative film.

As time passed, Roz realized that Paul was much more than a partier—that beneath the surface, they held the same values and dreams. When Paul asked Roz about whether or not she went to confession, she said, "Absolutely not. When I want to talk to God, I go directly to the Source." Paul was impressed by her solid sense of self, integrity, and faith. He grew to respect Roz deeply, and still does today.

"When we attend reunions," Roz said, "people are often shocked that we're still together. We broke up so many times! I studied abroad during my junior year in Rome. They were ten golden, life-altering months that dramatically shifted my worldview while simultaneously igniting an inner passion for the arts and travel that deeply colors my life to this day. Meanwhile, Paul was somewhat lost, trying to find himself in the counterculture of San Francisco in the '60s. We struggled to connect when I returned, and it was rough going. We were coming from two different worlds. In November of that year, we were engaged, but I returned the ring three months later. It felt like we'd arrived at an impasse. Thankfully, time apart helped us realize what we had, and after a lot of hard work, we were joyfully and confidently married in August of 1969. It was one hard-won commitment."

Three months later, when a twenty-two-year-old Roz became pregnant while on the pill, Paul and Roz were forced to grow up fast. Something in Paul said, "Rise up."

After over fifty years of marriage, they look back over the decades with an abiding sense of respect for one another. Roz claims, "We always go to the mat together." Their capacities to talk, laugh, forgive, extend compassion, and hold one another accountable are the practices that keep them together. Paul and Roz's relationship testifies to their stamina for taking on challenges from the very beginning.

When they met, Paul and Roz were both devoted yet questioning Catholics. While their fidelity to a spiritual path never wavered, it led them down many unexpected roads and detours, searching for an authentic spiritual life they could embrace. Like many of our generation, their college years were defined by a fierce, open-minded approach to questioning and rejecting long-held traditions. While in Rome, Roz witnessed first-hand the excesses and abuses of power in the Vatican, ground zero for Roman Catholicism. She found herself unsettled, having little to hang on to in terms of her faith.

Meanwhile, with his outgoing nature, Paul was drawn to the Jesus Movement that was popular in the late '60s and early '70s, where new forms of faith communities were explored. Paul described the group as close-knit and one where he made a strong confession of faith. He characterized this experience as "wonderful and cultish," as it addressed his need for belonging. Looking back, Paul valued this time as a beneficial chapter in his journey. Because of his youth, he overlooked some red flags, particularly concerning gender issues and rigid rules. Drawn to combining alternative lifestyles with new methods of worship, the baby boomer generation often made great sacrifices of time and treasure to participate in these communities. Many cults subsequently flourished in this exciting "new age" of spiritual and social reform.

Although Roz tasted potential in Paul's new church, she was wary. Head coverings for women were strongly encouraged and participation in "worldly events" was discouraged.

Paul soon became an elder, while Roz never quite felt at home. They were members of this community for ten years. They recounted these as lean financial years when they rented out their newly purchased first home in San Jose so they could help establish a new church in Berkeley. Paul realized that he was looking for a sense of belonging he'd missed in his childhood. The church provided this up to a point. He was encouraged to develop his gifts for speaking and leadership. Roz, meanwhile, was led in a different direction. She focused on nurturing a keen inner life, a quest that started in earnest while living in Rome. As their children grew, Paul and Roz began to question the health of this community for their family, especially concerning gender issues. They left the church in the mid '80s.

Burnt out from this experience, Paul and Roz threw themselves into their time with their children, careers, and community. Then, in 1994, Paul came into a season of crisis when his mother was dying, and old scars from unresolved childhood wounds began to haunt him. He felt he needed the "word of God" back in his life. Again, he committed to a church near their home, where he eventually became an elder. Roz, always more cautious about church communities, hung back. "Again, I resisted," she said, "in light of the painful experiences from the past. In time, however, predicated on the positive change I saw in Paul, I joined him at this new church. And gradually, my heart was warmed. I began to serve and was invited into an external Bible study, where later I was called into leadership. We were active in this church for a decade, assuming various roles and ministries. While on a church-sponsored trip to Israel, we were invited to help plant a new church for the next generation, where we could serve as mentors and help young couples prepare for marriage. Sadly, this experience, while brief, also ended painfully."

Paul and Roz then returned to their neighborhood church. Entering his mid-fifties, Paul responded to an invitation to join the pastoral team. "I took a leap of faith and stepped out of a thirty-year career in banking and financial management to assume that position. Financially, it was a gamble. My role was to act as a liaison between the pastoral team and the elders. Unfortunately, dysfunction and rigidity comprised a large part of this system, which I did not fully appreciate going in. It was a difficult and frustrating season. I was trying to affect change in an organization with little room for movement. Eventually, the church ruptured. In the end, I was outspoken and addressed the community. I didn't make many friends with the old guard leadership that night, but the congregation broke out in applause when they heard the straight story. Still, I came away broken-hearted; it was clear we were done."

During these years, Paul addressed his shadows and childhood wounds in therapy. "There came a point when I knew I had to do deeper interior work when I could no longer suppress childhood issues. My therapist was truthful and piercingly tough, just what I needed. It was hard, painful work, but slowly I began to change. I got healthier and freer. I was in psychotherapy for seven years, learning to get out of my head and feel. I found my voice, power, and our marriage and family life reaped the benefits."

It is not always easy to distinguish our spiritual needs from our psychological issues. Indeed, it is probably a false dichotomy to oppose them. As Saint Teresa of Ávila's work on the mansions of the soul highlights, humans have "reptiles" in our lower mansions from growing up in the human condition, formed unconsciously in childhood with imperfect parents. James Finley calls these wounds and unresolved trauma "the cross we must bear." Whatever you call them, we can't bypass our wounds spiritually by losing ourselves in service and devotional practices. They catch up with us, as they did for Paul, and we must face them directly, often with help from a therapist, spiritual director, or both. It is not unusual for this to happen later in life, for as we slow down, our shadows find us.

Roz added, "This process stirred up Paul's pain. It was hard to watch, but I was impressed with his courage. My respect for him grew. Before therapy, he wasn't always present. He was often there, but not. That pattern began to fade once he dug in and did the work."

After many years and many churches, numerous starts and stops, joys and disappointments, Paul and Roz finally embraced a more contemplative spirituality in their sixties. They each sought out spiritual directors and began to attend local contemplative retreats, focusing on their spiritual formation. It wasn't long before they enrolled in seminary to be trained as spiritual directors. Today, they both serve pastors in the greater Bay Area.

With age a natural change occurs, marked by a stronger inward pull toward our depths, more silence, and solitude. Paul said, "My priorities have shifted. I spent years working in the church and am now serving outside of it. I want less activity, more silence, and solitude. Intentionally, I am slowing down; that is where life is. I am also exploring other avenues, particularly poetry and art. Roz and I take advantage of the many cultural and contemplative offerings at Stanford University, near our home. And I thoroughly enjoy spending more time with our children and nine grandchildren."

Roz reflected similar sentiments. "Solitude is where I draw my energy. This place, our home, is a sanctuary. By design, we maintain a quiet pace. God is leading me to honor my limitations and embrace my desires. My spiritual direction practice reflects that call; it always brings me life. It is particularly rewarding as I see my one-on-one meetings with pastors create a ripple effect in their communities."

Paul concluded, "I believe we take this calm interiority out into the world, starting each morning with a good hour to meditate, read and pray. Then we carry that peace into our days."

Paul and Roz know they are blessed in sharing these inner life desires. Their spirituality is what drew them together in the first place.

We asked Paul and Roz about their most challenging experience. They both named a lawsuit from which they were still recovering. "We were embroiled in a family lawsuit that lasted for four years," Paul explained. "My father-in-law left a sizable estate his second family challenged. We made multiple attempts to settle with them, to no avail. It was a grueling, energy-draining process involving dozens of lawyers. And yet, by God's grace, we learned to hold things lightly."

"Our litigator encouraged us to go to trial," Roz added, "but it wasn't worth it to sacrifice any further distraction from our precious lives. Ironically, in the end, the case was settled in mediation, and I received exactly what my dad intended."

As they discussed this painful experience, it was clear Roz and Paul learned much in the process. Spiritually, they honed their values over the long duration of this lawsuit and chose to live well and endure. Because it spanned a four-year period, they had to hold the tension, make the most of their lives, and trust the experience without compromising their integrity. Roz explained, "We came together every morning for Centering Prayer, grounding us for the day ahead." Paul added, "A lot of pain is caused by not accepting what is. Buoyed by the grace of God and the prayer of friends, we faced each day head-on."

Many of us become entangled in long, drawn-out struggles at work, in our families, and in our society, as we are experiencing now. Paul and Roz offer an example of using these times for growth. They developed character and grew closer, whereas some couples might have been torn apart. They not only survived but thrived. As witnessed in these interviews, sometimes our "worst of times" in the outer world become the "best of times" on a soul level.

Included in their list of challenges are health concerns. With the same openness with which they faced the lawsuit, they approached health issues as well. Paul disclosed, "Prostate cancer was a setback that knocked me out of my church role for six weeks. On Sunday morning I was always the guy that greeted, welcomed, and made announcements. Suddenly, all that was taken away. I tried to resurrect that guy when I recovered, but I couldn't find him. The timeout helped me see this."

This illness offered Paul a break from his routine and role at his church, creating a forced sabbatical. Like what we experienced in the pandemic, disease creates a natural incubation time for going within, realigning priorities, and breaking from old patterns, then returning in a new way—the eternal cycle of change. James Hillman, in his book *The Force of Character: And the Lasting Life*, advocates that instead of seeing the illnesses accompanying aging as failures or conditions to endure or hide, we should learn to read the information they contain.

> Dumbed down by our ideal of aging and the old wise person, we miss the forming of character that is actually taking place in these "symptoms" of aging. For that is where the wisdom lies . . .
> A body is a citadel of metaphors that can be

> read for psychological intelligence as well as bio-information. Look for the intelligence in the symptom. The body is a source of insight, to be read for its intelligence.[1]

Cancer eats up our cells and life source from within. Paul read his cancer diagnosis as an invitation to examine what, on the outside, might be depleting his life force. Within a year, he resigned both as an elder and a pastor.

Roz discussed a health challenge as well. "Five years ago, due to multiple joint replacements, I was home-bound for ten months. This changed the dynamics of our marriage. Both of my knees were replaced simultaneously, and then a few months later, my left hip required a revision to its initial replacement. Amid the recovery process, a complication arose that required exploratory surgery. As we waited for that surgery, we weren't sure if I would ever be able to walk unassisted again. Thankfully that issue was resolved, but throughout that season, Paul took on most household chores while also serving as my primary caregiver. So much was required of him!"

Like most of our couples, Paul and Roz witnessed their parents transition from this life. They considered the contrast they observed in each death, noticing how faith and fear impacted their parents' final days. As they recalled these experiences, they also reflected on what they desired for their own dying days.

"My mother's transition was laced with fear, for she had many unresolved issues," Paul said. "Toward the end, a priest visited her in the hospital. It was interesting to observe that peace triumphed over fear once she made her confession. In contrast, my aunt, a woman of deep faith, passed gently, peacefully."

Roz continued, "My parents died within seven months of one another. The disparity between their end-of-life experiences taught me a lot. A woman of faith, my mother entered hospice several months before she passed. When she first learned her time was limited, she smiled and said, 'I always wondered how I'd feel when I got here. What a nice surprise. I'm totally okay with this.' I watched a deep peace settle over her. She was so at ease, so ready. Then she thanked me for piping music into her hospital room. When I told her I had done no such thing, that I wasn't hearing anything, she just smiled and sang along, primarily to big band tunes from her youth. Soon I saw what was happening. Throughout her life, music was one of my mom's primary languages. I realized that our loving God was personally crafting her passage into the next life. On and off, those tunes visited her over the following weeks; always, she sang along."

She continued, "Once we knew she had about a day to live, the family gathered around her. As her breathing became more labored, a Threshold Choir arrived, courtesy of hospice, to help ease her passing with subtle chants. Before long, we watched her visibly relax as the music rolled over her. It seemed that she would pass soon, so we each expressed our love for her, and then I brought photos of departed loved ones before her eyes—her son, and her parents. 'They are waiting for you,' I said, and her gaze told me she agreed. The Celtic tradition calls this experience a thin place. I believe I was in that sacred space with my mother for months. Particularly at the end, it confirmed what I'd always known: there is no reason to fear death."

"On the other hand," Roz said, "my father had not followed much of a spiritual path. Watching him struggle and resist his death was not pretty, leading me to presume that we truly do die how we live. The contrast between these two experiences speaks to me still, which I treasure as an invaluable gift."

We asked Paul and Roz to elaborate on their thoughts about their own deaths, and their wisdom impressed us. While many couples we interviewed hadn't thought much about their deaths, Paul and Roz were not among them.

Paul began. "While I don't know what it will look like and am not anxious to get there, I believe in the mystery of eternal life. Even though I don't spend a lot of time thinking about it, I am curious."

Roz added, "That's exactly where I am. I believe we have an opportunity to experience life and death right now. Every day there is an invitation to die to ourselves. Learning to keep death before me is worth its weight in gold, for it helps me appreciate life in the moment. I also notice that holding both together is becoming more comfortable. And so, as we considered our move a few years ago, it only made sense that we find a one-story home with adequate space for a potential caregiver."

The notion of practicing for death, or keeping one's death in mind, is not a new one. We experience many "mini" deaths throughout life. In the Celtic tradition, there is a saying, "Die before you die." Paul and Roz are people openly discussing, facing, and preparing for the changes aging brings while also living vibrantly in the present.

We often ended our interviews with legacy questions, and on this note we conclude this chapter with this remarkable couple. Paul and Roz, deeply dedicated to their family, emphasized their love and value of family as their most significant legacy.

Roz began, "Legacy is an important word to me. My parents valued achievement. Yet when delivering their eulogies, their accomplishments were not my primary focus. I spoke of my father's lavish generosity. I spoke of the strength of my mother's faith that sustained her in trials and had a lasting impact on those she knew. When I consider our legacy, I trust that our faith and the path of perseverance through difficulties will influence those whose lives we've touched. Our kids know the struggles Paul went through and are proud of him for working as hard as he did—breaking the cycle for future generations. On its own, that is one powerful legacy."

Our presence is the legacy our children and friends will remember. From this interview, we carry a lasting image of Paul and Roz as courageous, faith-based seekers and pilgrims, persistent and strong in the face of their shadows and challenges, a couple who knew early on how to "go to the mat together." We are so grateful to and for them.

A GRACE NOTE

We are sad to share that Roz died from pancreatic cancer on December 8, 2021, after six months of illness. During her transition, she awoke from a coma to speak her final words. When we asked Paul for permission to include them in this chapter, he said that when asked by a hospice chaplain what Roz wanted to teach others with her dying, she said she wished to educate others about how to be intentional in preparing for and surrendering to death. In that spirit, we quote their daughter Eliza's account of Roz's final words, which she posted on Facebook.

"Four hours into her sedation, Mom unexpectedly came out of unconsciousness for about five minutes and had much to say. It was something special, incredible to witness, and a gift we all feel we should be more than okay with us sharing. Through labored breath and her sweet last smiles . . . here is some of what she had to say.

'What a way to go. WHAT A WAY TO GO. Everyone should be able to go like this. God is so good, you guys. I am so at peace. I hope you all have a death like this. So comfortable.

I feel so cared for. I am fighting nothing. Lucky me. God is good. There is nothing to fear. All is Light. Love is all there is. LOVE is all there is. This feels like being reborn. I am ready. I married so well. Paul Dumesnil, you have been a saint. I love you. I know the world can be hard and troubled but don't fall for it. All that matters is love. Do not let darkness blur your light. I will stay close. This connection we share. It cannot be lost.'"

We can be redeemed only to the extent to which we see ourselves.

MARTIN BUBER

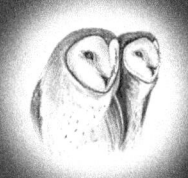

Blessed is the couple who
listens deeply to each other,
for they shall be seen,
understood, and met.

BLESSED IS THE COUPLE WHO
Listens Deeply to Each Other

INTRODUCING
STEVE & FAYE ORTON SNYDER

YEARS AGO, WHEN Faye and I were working on a writing project together, she happened to be visiting Jay and me in Bend, Oregon. At the time, she was dating Steve, whom she portrayed as someone who was (among many other things) a partner in an international law firm in San Francisco with her ex-husband, Luther, and a family friend of fifty-two years. Faye had been good friends with Steve's wife, Judy, and their children all knew each other. Years ago, Luther came to Steve with the news that he had decided to leave Faye. Luther tried to justify his decision and explain his feelings and the reasons for them. Steve defended the value of the marital bond, even under stress, and pointed out the rewards of taking the "road less traveled" in these situations. He argued that both Faye and Luther were exceptional people.

As you can probably guess, Luther didn't follow Steve's advice, and Faye was left on her own to raise their three children, complete her seminary studies, and launch her ministry as a Disciples of Christ pastor. Once her children were grown, Faye married a man named Mike, her church's choir director; it was only three years before he died suddenly of appendicitis. Years later, when Judy also died suddenly of a heart attack, Steve reached out to Faye for support for his grief. Within a year, they realized a growing attraction to one another.

One day while working on our project, Faye and I were hiking in the golden California hills surrounding her home in Lafayette, near San Francisco. As we marched up the trail, we were knocking around ideas for the program's title when Faye blurted out, "How about 'The Geography of Grace'?" Of course, the title landed. Looking back, it seemed to name the landscape of her and Steve's relationship as well, a geography of grace.

Years later, we sat in the same cozy home in Lafayette, interviewing Steve and Faye about the story of what brought them together and what has kept them together. From Faye's earlier visit to Bend, we recalled how much she admired Steve as the most brilliant, intelligent person she had ever met, one of rock-solid integrity, curiosity, depth, humor, and loyalty. Jay and I secretly wondered how that image had held up over time, now seven years into their marriage, and were pleasantly surprised that the answer was "splendid." However, back in Bend, she never could have imagined the many challenges that lay ahead for them.

There is often an element of mystery as to why people are attracted to each other. At their ages, both Steve and Faye were highly accomplished leaders in their respective fields of law and ministry. They were in the process of retiring, relaxing their hard-earned identities and successes in the world, and turning toward home. Among other things, Faye and Steve held in common a geography of grief as widow and widower.

Faye described herself as being pastoral when she initially began seeing Steve. He was in the early stages of loss, asking himself, "What will happen to me?" One night they sat outside for eight hours drinking wine and realized that they wanted to be together.

Steve portrayed those early days as follows. "My wife, Judy, had just died, and we had been married thirty-nine years. Faye's second husband, Mike, [had] died seven years ago, and she was back on her feet, but I was out of balance. In the process of talking to everyone I knew who had lost a spouse, I asked, 'Is there life beyond this tunnel?' I started to go to Faye's every Tuesday, where she gave me a bowl of soup and an ear. She put her arms around me and comforted me in a way that helped me balance again. Within a year, I had fallen in love with her. Here was a wonderful woman who considered spending the rest of her life with me. We had frank talks, being honest about our health challenges, our feelings, and what we wanted, which painted a picture of the togetherness I had hoped for in marriage. Faye was always honest and forthright—what she says, you can take to the bank. I got her with the motor home. One of my dreams was to get married, tour the country in a motor home, and this was one of her dreams too."

Their relationship is a compelling example of what a couple can experience later in life, post-career, after the intense responsibilities of raising young children. Faye and Steve sensed the potential in front of them and grabbed on to this opportunity.

Steve continued, "The word 'wholesome' comes to mind. The deeper I fell in love with Faye, the more light came into my world. I felt restored to my youth and turned back the clock to places I hadn't dreamed possible for me. I was grateful for her attentive and empathic listening and concern. I felt euphoric at that time, but not naïve because I knew her so well. She used to go on our vacations after Mike died. I could see her pain and ability to bear up under tough circumstances. She is a truly centered person who deals with loss. I was not through with mourning. Faye assured me I would get through it just as she had with Mike and that she would be there for me as long as I wished it."

As we listened to them, we were struck by how much this couple respected and admired each other. A strong fabric of common values holds them together. In their presence, you know you are with people who are "the salt of the earth." Because they were blending two very different families, they immediately encountered many challenges that forced them to clarify and embody these values. They encountered severe health concerns, including Faye's need for two knee replacements, Steve's heart attack, and his fall in the shower that led to knee surgery (reattachment of a detached quadriceps tendon). He also underwent back surgery, a product of his time in the infantry, daily carrying fifty-plus pounds of gear and weaponry on a 150-pound frame, mile after mile, in the Annamese highlands of Vietnam. In other words, next to their excitement about this fresh beginning in a new marriage, they weren't naïve regarding what it would take to come to terms with their aging. One of their stated values was caring for their health. Faye and Steve promised each other they would not deny, hold back, or turn away from things they were concerned about regarding their physical conditions. They would not be judgmental, but supportive.

Another of their mutual values is the belief in putting family first. Faye has three adult children, while Steve has four, one of whom was killed in 2014. Their current grandchild count is eighteen, with nine girls and nine boys. Their family takes up significant time and attention. They change their calendars when their kids need them and enjoy what Faye calls "good exhaustion" from taking care of and entertaining their brood.

Their vows to harbor no secrets, exercise courage by facing problems directly, and seek help as needed came into play when Faye and Steve encountered certain problematic realities. They had to decide what it meant to blend families with adult children who were raised with disparate rules, values, and norms and were still haunted by the memories of deceased or divorced spouses.

Faye disclosed how she initially sought counseling for help with stepmothering. "We went to a therapist, older than us, a very wise lady. We presented our high expectations for our relationship and our need to delve into this. We met with her for quite a while to launch this relationship. She was brilliant. She would say a line, and I still carry those lines in me. For instance, 'The role of stepmother is the most impossible role in society.' That is true. She would say, 'Let's see all that is here.' She gave us help to do that. I had to know, in the beginning, if I mattered as much and more than his kids. I railed against things with his kids I felt I didn't have any power over. I wasn't a player in any of it, feeling more like an observer rather than a participant. I was lost. I have boundary issues that got stirred up from my upbringing. I felt my boundaries on how to be as a family were solid, but Steve's kids didn't know about them. For instance, I wondered, 'Why didn't they help clean up after dinner? Why did they sit and want me to wait on them?' That doesn't feel right. I was angry. We were trying to soft-peddle to them, to make them feel welcome here. They had recently lost their mother. This struggle was partly me, partly them, and partly us; we eventually figured it out. I felt like a step-monster. There was so much hidden I couldn't describe. I needed to know for sure that Steve was on my side. But I paradoxically got to see who

I really am. That is a gift that keeps on giving." What a great example of how grace appears in dark places.

Ironically, in life, when claiming a value or ideal like 'family is important,' we encounter roadblocks within ourselves to embody it, as Faye experienced with Steve's adult children. These challenges usually represent our growth edges. Faye and Steve's strength as a couple is in exercising the courage to face problems and tensions head-on, seek help, and take the time to address these concerns. A healthy couple values their relationship so highly that they work on it, learn new skills, and seek the truth and support. It often entails unlearning old, anti-relational habits. The gift Faye received through their therapy was finding her inner strength and integrity to work through this difficult situation of step-parenting. Love requires good boundaries and strong self-esteem. She was pushed in both areas and emerged with an enhanced sense of agency.

Steve also encountered some old and unconscious anti-relational habits that worked against his capacity to be intimate with Faye. When he withdrew into his familiar, isolated world of working and writing in his study, Faye called him out for more engagement with her. He had never been with someone who expected his full presence. Steve had to learn to show up; he reported he is now profoundly grateful for this. Steve's willingness to be influenced by Faye is an example of how relationships transform. When we are willing to listen to each other deeply, and change our behaviors when they hurt our partners or interfere with intimacy, relationships can thrive.

Both Steve and Faye each encountered deep wells of grief many times in their lives. Steve was exposed to an overwhelming amount of death as a young man when drafted during the Vietnam War, where he served as a lieutenant infantry officer in "D" (Delta) Company of the 1st Battalion 9th Marines regiment (known as the "1/9"), Third Marine Division. The 1/9 is famously known in the Marine Corps as "The Walking Dead," named in part for its high rate of casualties during four years (1965–1969) of service, featured in the documentary *The Vietnam War*, by Ken Burns and Lynn Novick. Steve served with the "Walking Dead" from July '66 to July '67. During the four years of combat in Vietnam, about 750 of 1/9's marines or sailors were killed in action.

Steve was scheduled for a screening interview for the Ken Burns film, during which time he broke down emotionally and realized he couldn't participate. He still carries in his valise a list of the names of each person, written in his minuscule script, all 747 killed in his unit, and remembers them regularly. He showed this list to us with tears in his eyes. Perhaps we would all be wise to keep the names of our lost ones in our wallets, for not all relationships end with death. Grief is not something to fix or forget, but to carry. Steve does this out of respect for them and for honoring an overwhelming, unfathomable, and absurd amount of death that the war brought to him (and our generation). Steve realized death isn't something to "get over" but to integrate and hold its mystery near his heart. We sincerely appreciated his candor, for many people are married to veterans who bear the trauma and memories of war to their graves.

As a minister, Faye often worked with the dying and benefitted from her unique upbringing. "I grew up hearing death framed as a joyful thing. I was reared in a bedrock of fundamentalism. My parents are buried together, feet facing east. They believed they would stand up in the last call and live anew in heaven. My father was a chaplain in a poor house, so I saw him preside over deaths with great joy, for he believed the people living there would be better off. When my ministry took me to so many dying people, watching them cross over, I again saw the joy. Several came back and told the story. They reported crossing over a threshold that contained joy, peace, and relief. Perhaps there is another dimension I would welcome too. We just don't know. However, I am not scared but curious, and I will be telling myself in my last days, 'I want to do this with grace. I want to be known for not being a victim but for my acceptance of death. I want to be allowing for what is going to be to become.' I imagine myself buttoning up my coat and leaving quietly."

None of these experiences with death protected them from the shock of losing one of their children. Steve disclosed what happened to his daughter, Karen, who was staying in a resort motel in Fort Bragg on the coast in Mendocino County, California, taking care of her sister's crying baby. Next door to her was a man enraged by the noise and who ran his truck into her room through the plate glass window. Karen managed to save the infant by tossing her on the bed but could not save herself. "She was murdered. There was no warning. It is unexplainable, but this guy ran her over with a truck. It was evil. The pain and anguish put a lot of stress on us, and we wondered how we would continue to manage things. Could our love survive? It did. It is hard to describe how painful this truly was."

Part of what complicated the situation, as mentioned earlier, was that Faye and Steve were establishing rules for their new home and space as a blended family. Faye struggled to create boundaries that could work for her as she welcomed Steve's children's visits. Karen was someone who had a hard time changing and adjusting to the rules.

Steve said, "Karen's death was like pulling the bottom orange out from the stack of our family culture. She was that powerful of a force in holding us together. As the eldest child, she was uncompromising in her values and went out of her way to care for others in the family, like her uncle Joe or her grandmother.

The circumstances of her death provide a good example. She had driven the three-and-a-half hours to Fort Bragg the day before she was killed to care for her sister's seven-month-old baby so her sister could go out with friends."

Faye added, "For Steve, his family culture was not regimented, but like a bunch of puppies rolling down a hill together; his wife, Judy, managed everything. People came and went as they willed and didn't clean up after themselves. Karen was unique, honest, direct, and deeply committed to the family, but transgressed the house rules we were establishing. She expected you to do for her as she would do for you. She was killed in the midst of us working on these issues.

"I look back and wish I had known more about Karen's limits, and what she needed. Karen needed the feeling of home, being held, being worth something, and being affirmed as a mother. I didn't catch on. We have survived but are still grieving, and it still washes over us. It is always here and always will be. There is now an empty chair at the table. You don't get over it; you learn how to carry it. I know I didn't respond to her as compassionately as I wish. All I can do now is deeply listen to the pain."

Given all of these stories that brought to light their trials, we asked them, "When do you feel most loved by the other?"

Steve began, "I am a tactile person. I don't know how I got that way. Mom would tell me stories of rubbing my back. With my back surgery, I had lots of nerve pain down my legs into my feet—shooting, burning pains. Every night, Faye walks in, rubs my feet, puts me to bed, walks around, turns off the light, takes my glasses off, and I am in heaven. I know how much I am loved. These are tiny pieces of devotion that keep the train on track. Faye also has the gifts of spiritual and emotional discernment and language to express them. I live in deep dark places. The war, loss of Karen, my work, and the more trying periods of my thirty-nine years of marriage to Judy, all live in these places. Faye is pastor emeritus and helps to rebuild me. I feel loved and that I am not such a bad person after all."

Then Faye responded. "I most feel loved when Steve can witness my pain. When I ask him to see me through my angst, and when he can hang in there long enough to get it all from me, I feel loved. He just doesn't move. I have never had this in my life. My Dad was emotionally unavailable, so I learned warmth from my faith community but never lived with it close to home. Steve's ability to hear my frustration about him being stuck in his office and unavailable to me is an example of this. He is the perfect receptacle to put in the raw stuff. He doesn't move. It gives me total trust that I will be fine. I realize, 'You can do this.' He uses few words but serves as a witness and deep listener. I feel loved witnessing the generosity of his spirit towards me, the world, friends, family, and work. He gives more than he takes. He works hard and gives it all. He is a container that can hold for me, so very mature. This is the real deal. When I am truly seen, I am known and loved. He takes time and effort to know me."

Communication serves up the daily bread of relationships. Steve cherishes Faye's physical contact and care of his body and her loving attention when in discernment. Faye appreciates Steve's capacity to witness her pain, hear her, see her, and in these ways, feel known and loved.

Jay and I were curious how two accomplished, career-oriented people found meaning and purpose in retirement. Both revealed how they each discovered surprising creative endeavors. Steve said, "I enjoyed writing the family memoir with Judy, which turned out 1,300 pages long. It was a genealogy. Some parts that describe the family were circulated among all of the cousins and were met with an outcry of anger and distress, all part of the price honesty demanded. That was a burst of creativity. All those words, I can't take any of them back. I want to do more of that. It would be great to work on a small-town newspaper at a local level."

Faye also discovered some new creative directions. "I backed into a passion when our house started, literally, going downhill. It was sliding off its foundation! We, therefore, also did some significant, necessary remodeling. I discovered that I loved working with contractors and had a clear idea of what I wanted it to become. I always liked designing and decorating the home with pillows, dishes, tables, and all things associated with the home. I have a deep passion for hospitality and taking care of others. I didn't have it as a child, being cared for like this. Things weren't nice for me. Now you can take me anywhere, and I will rearrange things and make them mine. The overriding passion is creating a home. This is a baseline for me."

As we age, our priorities can change dramatically and often show up as a surprising loss of energy and interest in activities, social engagements, and people who were once considered important. We asked Faye and Steve the question, "What do you no longer have energy for, and that now feels like a waste of time?"

Faye said, "Cocktail parties are feeling like a waste of time! Before I say yes, I ask, 'What will go on there?' Tennis groups, any group; I just don't get energy there. Now I am drawn to smaller settings and am more interested in picking up some Chinese food and talking with a few people."

"I've had trouble going back to the church after retiring," Faye added. "I don't need to be there, even though they love it when I come. I am not in and not out, but I don't know as many people anymore. We have been involved with the Marines, with the people struggling with PSTD and death. Now *that* is real and is still one group we maintain a relationship with, but it has decreased since Steve is not in a leadership role. Give me three people on my front porch. I am not lamenting that I don't belong to big groups. I don't want to."

Steve reflected, "Over the years, I was involved with scouting, the YMCA, the Marines Memorial, and homeless veterans. I helped with the Danny Foundation, which focused on nursery safety, and I felt as though I was engaged and contributing. I don't feel I am contributing anymore, and see there are smarter and younger people doing this work. I am pulling back and making way for them. This is my last year for these things. This doesn't mean I won't do something in the future, but I need to get closer to home to resolve legacy issues and come up with something Faye and I can do together. I have dropped the ball in the area of politics, which we will take a serious look at. The civics courses are not doing a good job. I fault the school boards and their limited budgets. If you love this country, you have to be serious about developing citizenship and ownership. I don't see this happening. Those who have served in our military are no longer represented as fully as they once were in the body politic, for example, after WWII."

Finally, we invited Faye and Steve to discuss their inner lives and how they pursue their spiritual interests at this stage of life. Steve began, "I need my alone time, but that is not the right description. My alone time happens whether I need it or not. We carry a pack of historical things we are processing at this age. One great benefit of a relationship later in life is helping each other by creating space and then being there to witness, but not interfere with those processes."

Faye also needs alone time. "With the whirlwind from family, there is a point [when] I am exhausted. I have to claim some quiet and be by myself. I like to reflect on life, to savor our lives, and I need to have the time to think about meaning.

I ask, 'Where was meaning today?' That comes through journaling, sitting, and being still. I wish I had been doing this all along, savoring my life. It has been beautiful and good. But I better practice this before getting into my eighties. I am calling myself to pay attention and take the time to go deeper. I get tears when I realize how fortunate we are, and how much love has passed through this house. There is nothing like long walks by myself. These alone times are not just life-giving but life-preserving for me. I could do more of that."

We conclude their narrative with one final story about Steve and Faye's adventures. While we were discussing our plans to set forth on a cross-country trip in our RV to interview the rest of the couples for *Side by Side*, we asked them if they were still taking trips in their motor home. Faye recounted their mishap on their final motorhome trip, where they got a late start on a drive on Interstate 5 next to Mt. Shasta in their brand-new Winnebago. Steve was too tired to drive, so he went in back to sleep, and Faye took over. However, she fell asleep at the wheel and they awoke to the tumult of their RV rolling over on the highway. It was totaled, but by the grace of God, no one was hurt. They decided not to replace the RV—it was time to cease traveling in this fashion. We can't help but picture this couple protected by angels, two survivors and thrivers through difficult times, and who continue to live together, side by side in a geography of grace. We feel so blessed to know them.

I do not at all understand the mystery of grace—
only that it meets us where we are
but does not leave us where it found us.

ANNE LAMOTT

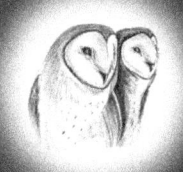

Blessed is the couple who
practices compassion,
for they shall honor the
Spark of the Divine in all of
their brothers and sisters.

BLESSED IS THE COUPLE WHO
Practices Compassion

INTRODUCING
BOBBY BELLAMY & BARBARA BLAIN-BELLAMY

WE STOPPED FOR lunch on our way to meet Barbara and Bobby in downtown Conway, where Barbara proudly serves as the first Black mayor in all of South Carolina. A thriving, tourist-friendly historic river town established in 1732, we learned it currently has around 23,000 residents. Ambling down the walkway along the Waccamaw River, which is lined with live oak trees, we came across a vibrant, crowded bistro full of professionals enjoying a creative, gourmet menu that could rival big-city restaurants.

After lunch, Jay and I pulled onto a quiet street and parked in front of their brick home. Hauling our film equipment up the pathway, their door flew open, and we were greeted with warm, welcoming hugs, one of the signatures of this couple. Barbara's tight schedule commanded us to focus, with only three of the usual six hours for the interview. We instantly dropped into a deep conversation.

While they married later in life, Bobby and Barbara had known each other since young adulthood. As Barbara put it, they didn't have a very good beginning. She recounts an incident from a party when she was married to Bobby's high school friend and, in her words, they were young and lacked good sense. Upon returning home, her then-husband told Barbara that Bobby said he was surprised that he had married her. Bobby had made fun of her posture and the fact that she was pigeon-toed. She never forgot the sting of his words and noted that she had much earlier corrected her posture by walking around with a stack of books on her head. Later in life, they met again, and she confronted Bobby about his criticism. He denied having said such a thing. While she didn't believe him, she did finally forgive him. Their lives were connected in other ways too. Bobby's sister was Barbara's good friend, and his mother had, for over thirty years, been her seamstress. Encounters between Bobby and Barbara were sporadic, but they happened upon each other every year or so.

Bobby built a career in the Air Force, where he served US presidents and dignitaries on Air Force One, earning the highest rank attainable by an enlisted airman directing a logistics team charged with air delivery. He retired as a Chief Master Sergeant after twenty-seven years of service. He had a brief marriage early in his life, with a son and daughter born into this union.

During those twenty-eight-plus years, Barbara earned an undergraduate degree, then worked for twenty-five years as a social worker focusing on child protection. A divorce ending an eighteen-year marriage opened her up to an interest in local government. Barbara landed a seat on the Conway City Council in the next election. At age forty-six, she went to law school. Later she worked as a prosecutor, a defense counsel, a counsel for her county's Department of Social Services handling child abuse cases, and managed a private practice, working with low-income clientele. Ten years after her divorce, she met and married a gentleman with whom she had a good life. He died suddenly from a heart attack before they could celebrate their tenth anniversary.

Barbara later met up with Bobby, whose fiancé had recently died of colon cancer. Since Barbara was a lawyer, Bobby approached her to help him with some legal issues. When she refused payment for her assistance, he invited her out to dinner. She didn't consider it a date, but she had lost thirty-five pounds since becoming a widow and realized that it might be pleasant to have dinner with a friend. Since it was mid-summer, the neighboring Myrtle Beach was full of tourists, and they couldn't get into a restaurant until 9 p.m. After the long wait, they enjoyed a leisurely meal, where Barbara soon realized that she had misjudged Bobby. Barbara saw Bobby as a free spirit. He had been married but divorced in the 1970s. Ever since, she had watched him and maintained that he was always a show-off with his fancy cars and string of pretty women on his arm. He was not to be taken seriously. However, spending time with him, she saw through her judgments and found a genuine sweetness and steady calmness in him. He walked her inside her home and kissed her on the cheek. That was the beginning of their current story, which they are still writing together. At the time of the interview, Barbara and Bobby had been married four years.

When we asked them what has kept them together, they didn't hesitate to name their commitment to each other, love of family, and faith backgrounds. Barbara noted, "I don't want to do this life alone. Aging and life can be pretty tough. There is nothing like having a person who is home to you, knows the best and worst in you, and cares anyway. I love having a home where I can collect myself, walk in the door, be overjoyed to be together, and share. When I became a widow, I was going to sell my house. I thought that I couldn't handle all that goes into maintaining it, dealing with tradespeople, scheduling, conflicts, etc. Bobby gets it done. He calls in a professional and writes a check. I get to focus on what is more critical in my world because he is taking care of the day-to-day. He also brings with him a whole new family. I have lost so many from my own family, and I have gained another mother. She genuinely likes me. She once told Bobby I was the smartest woman he knew. Bobby has a sister and children, and out of that long list, there is four-year-old Kennedy. I now have three sets of children and grandchildren. Kennedy is a sweet, precocious, fascinating little girl with a rich personality. Probably because Kennedy is our first grandchild to grow up here, I have learned a new degree of love."

Their love of family is a core value for them, yet they were both raised under challenging circumstances. Bobby never lets forty-eight hours pass without seeing his mother or catching up with his sister. He knows everyone's birthdays and children's names. While Barbara, at age sixty-seven, is still going 24/7 in her position as mayor, Bobby, at seventy-two, finds himself enjoying retirement years focused on relationships and adjusting to the physical changes with age. He values Barbara's role and takes supporting her seriously, treasuring the time they carve out together.

A tall, big bear of a quiet man, Bobby relishes his time alone and enjoys accompanying Barbara when needed. In his younger years, he was dedicated to and identified with sports, including running forty-five miles a week, playing football, riding bikes, playing golf, and so on. The physical changes and diminishment of these capacities with aging have been tough. At fifty-one, he developed a back problem and scaled back. He says, "I see life as stages: twenties, thirties, and now I am an old man. I am not entirely disabled but have slowed down quite a bit. I am almost bald, but I have pictures around that show how I used to look. I have learned to live with it. Age is a funny thing. I want to be around but I've had a full life. I notice these changes every five to seven years. Life is good."

When we asked him who he is, deep down, he claimed, "I am a fair person. I achieved E-9 status in the Air Force and made it early in my career by being fair with the ones above and below me. I am honest. I shared all the love I had inside of me. People describe me as dopey, playful, happy, and funny. But most importantly, trustworthy."

Although only six years younger, Barbara is at a different stage of life, going strong in the community. In her presence, her sparky energy and enthusiasm are contagious. She had a lot to say about the essence of her work in the world. "I am a spreader of hope. I live in a place and time when people struggle with so many issues. If there is one word I can direct thoughts and interests toward, it is hope. My effort is to teach children the personal value of self, and show them that they are full of nothing but potential. A small-town mayor may not be rated an exciting accomplishment by some, but it is huge for me. I grew up in Jim Crow-structured Conway, South Carolina. No one expected this honored position to be a part of my trajectory.

At every opportunity, I tell children of my humble beginnings, the value of curiosity, reading, and learning, and the enormity of people willing to help any dream come true. They should strive beyond the ordinary. When I am asked, as mayor, what we are doing about crime, I share that it is not about more officers or new weapons, body cameras, etc. I say to them, 'I volunteer twenty weeks a year at Conway Elementary, giving children what I believe they need to grow up to be proud, contributing, successful, good members of society. There is nothing better I can do about crime than that.'"

While naming herself a "spreader of hope," Barbara also owns that she has the heart of a teacher, and if she could, she would become an elementary educator. After retiring from her law career, she even looked into certification, but it would have taken two full years of schooling. She recalls her teachers believing in her and predicting she would do something meaningful. Becoming the first Black mayor in a town nestled in the Deep South is no small accomplishment. (Schools were not desegregated in Horry County until 1970.)

Barbara's faith guides her work in the world. She recalls a Sunday School teacher, Mrs. Bernice M. Johnson, who used to invent parables. One involved God sending Jesus to earth to check up on us. Barbara relayed Mrs. Johnson's lesson. "She said, 'I warn you, he will not wear a robe and sandals, a minister's robe, suit, or tie. He might be dirty, a little bit obnoxious, and get on your nerves. God might plant a little alcohol on his breath. Be careful how you treat people. You never know who might be Jesus.'"

Barbara continued, "I live among thousands of Jesus. I hope I honor them as though they are Jesus. We are not to judge people, which I have to work on."

She cited an example. "Recently, I was in a downpour in traffic. I had sat through a traffic light for three cycles when a woman stopped in front of me, exited the passenger door, weaved through two lanes of traffic, and seemed to be acting unreasonably. I am creating all kinds of stories regarding what this is about. Why can't she wait? I am making ugly judgments about this woman. Then she takes an interest in something on the ground, bends down, stands again to cross another lane, and walks onto a grassy hill. I see her clearly. She carefully places a baby turtle out of danger. I don't need to say any more. This puts me in my place. Accept people for who they are, where they are, and say things encouraging.

If I am a hoity-toity mayor, or a hoity-toity, judgmental human being, I diminish my value and am useless as the unofficial life coach I see myself being."

When we invited Bobby and Barbara to reflect on what has challenged their relationship, they quickly noted it had to do with family and how they have different approaches to caring for their granddaughter Kennedy. Our parenting styles are shaped by how we are parented. Based on how she was raised, Barbara approaches parenting authoritatively. She notes that her parents were in charge. In her words, "With our grandchild, I am consistently the adult. Whining and tears do not change our household rules. They are not harsh but clear. Teaching respect is my goal, not promoting fear. I give loads of praise, tenderness, and encouragement, but she is a little girl who is not ready for independence or authority. On a different side of the house, Bobby's style is accepting of all behaviors. He repeats what he tells her to do or not do, and she pays him little or no attention. She whimpers, and they're off to a store for another toy. I believe she sees her grandfather (Papa) as someone to manipulate.

"I call him passive and a pushover; he calls me a meanie. A parenting or grandparenting style where we find a middle ground is probably the goal. But for now, neither of us sees the logic in the other's methods. I pray the combination somehow helps her discover her ever-changing place in the world."

Bobby disclosed that during his childhood, his father left South Carolina and the family for Lancaster, Pennsylvania, to find work, and he was supposed to come back for his mom, but he never did; Bobby was raised mainly by his mother. "He would come home and go back, breaking my heart. By coming back four to five times a year, I never saw him for more than eight or nine days a year." His father's absence had a significant impact on his youth, and Bobby worked hard to forgive him. Later in life, when his dad had a stroke, his mom took his father back for the last seven years of his life. After his father died, Bobby said, "I had to let it go. I can honestly say it had a serious impact on me as a high school student and as a young man in the military, but I had to let it go. We will just leave it alone. I will leave it alone."

Barbara said, "My family was not particularly a good parenting model either. My mom became pregnant at sixteen, and my father married her. My dad is probably not my biological father, which adds to my love and admiration for him. I was spared this information for too long. I was his favorite. They were kids, forced to live together and be parents. They didn't get along or work well together. The poverty I lived in shouldn't have been that bad. Their inability to work and pull funds together hurt us. For instance, they argued over the electric bill. From their inability to agree on whose turn it was to pay the bill, the electricity would be turned off. By the time I was ten or twelve, I remember knowing they shouldn't be together. Each of them had leaned outside of marriage to give them a reason to smile. Living in a small town, we picked up on cues. When I consider the 1950s, what else was there to do but warm up together? They didn't have TV, football, movies, other activities, or outlets. It was just the way it was. I didn't learn relationship skills from my parents. Through God's grace, you learn to make decisions differently and want to give your children a nurturing environment. Nothing is more important than creating a better experience for the little people in your lives."

Their relationship with God is never far from the conversation and manifests itself in many dimensions of their lives. Bobby and Barbara share a Baptist religious background and practice many of its traditions, including tithing, regular prayers, attending church services, and following the Ten Commandments. Barbara reflects on her unique spiritual practice of hugging every person she encounters as an embodiment of seeing each human as a brother or sister; her hugs are a powerful form of extending love and mercy through each encounter. In her words, "Human touch has value in our lives. A baby fed and kept clean but not touched or spoken to will not thrive. Hugging is the whole symbolic piece about how we need each other, our interdependence, and our oneness."

Barbara may not know this, but there is a living Indian Hindu guru (Mātā Amritānandamayī Devī, often known simply as Amma or "Mother"), who is revered as "the hugging saint" by her followers. Her motherly embrace is known as *Darshan*. She whispers in your ear, "My daughter, my daughter, my daughter" (or son) while embracing you, and in so doing, affirming all humans are family. Like Barbara, she is a spreader of hope.

Bobby highlighted his faith origins. "I was converted at an early age, at about fourteen, when I first found God. We had a revival meeting; a preacher asked us, the unsaved, to get down on our knees and ask God to forgive our sins. I accepted Jesus as my Savior at this meeting. I believe in God, pray, and all the things a Christian does. When I married Barbara, I joined her church. She is very religious. I enjoy church. I believe in heaven, and some of us on earth are living in it now. I believe that at death, you go to sleep and wake up to the fire and the judgment, and you will be judged and go from there. I will get to heaven."

Barbara noted, "I was born to people who were strong believers, whom I prayed for and with my entire life. I believe all good things come from God, and I am to be grateful to Him for His goodness. I don't understand not believing.

It is fundamental to my being. How did you get here? Look at a flower. Nothing can parallel God in His wisdom, His goodness, and His power. I couldn't marry a nonbeliever. Spirituality is deep in my being."

Her spiritual practice of hugging everyone also tested their relationship. She explains, "Here is a funny story. When we were first dating, Bobby noticed I hug all people. What he noticed was me hugging men. He brought it to my attention, and I understood it had meaning to him. I said to him, 'We need to talk about this. I love you and want to make things work for us. Some adjustments I am willing to make, but this is not one of them. This is who I am. I gain my energy from the cheek of another. Hugging people, I cannot and will not change. You'll have to get yourself another mate if you cannot live with it.' Now he limits this complaint to once or twice a year.

"I don't play with God, but I am fully invested in His service, goodness, and love, and I have every responsibility to tell people where this comes from," she continued. "I believe my future depends on my reverence, requests for forgiveness, and hope for a world beyond this one. I experienced that God picked me up and gave me hope in grievous times. I sat in church after becoming a widow, being so bitter, and thinking how I wished I hadn't awakened that morning. I sat on the back pew, wishing I was dead. God didn't give up on me. He stayed with me until I got to a place of reverence."

Closer to home, they have their granddaughter, Kennedy, lead them in prayer before each meal. Barbara elaborates, "We pray together, and when we walk around our home, it is not uncommon at all to say 'Lord have mercy,' which means so many things. The bottom line is an acknowledgment of God's presence, love, and power. When there is anything we can't grasp or control, we request His intervention. This is where we are opening our minds and clearing the air. We don't always go to bed at the same time. We often pray alone at bedtime and try to instill this in Kennedy. We want her to walk out our door with a prayer: that she has a good day, that people are friendly to her, and she is friendly to them; we teach things like that."

Barbara continued, "It is amazing how you pick up something good to promote your spirituality, and then you give it up. I was thirty years old and bought lunch in a fast-food restaurant. Once I began eating, an older gentleman, a stranger (maybe Jesus), gently scolded me for failing to offer thanks to my Father for my food, saying, 'You look like someone who knows better than to eat without thanking the Lord.' He was right. Now, food cannot be had without thanking God for it. That reminder was all I needed. When I get corrected, it gives me heart and puts me back where I am meant to be."

While we were cherishing this conversation for how it lifted up the beauty of practicing a traditional Christian life so faithfully, we were soon delighted to hear about other dimensions of their spirituality when we asked them about mystical experiences. Listening to Barbara, we might have been, again, at the feet of a Hindu mystic.

"I think of a mystical experience as one beyond what is ordinary, even unexplainable, like an out-of-body experience, or knowing something we cannot justify knowing. For instance, when I experience a place I think I have visited before, like déjà vu, but it was more than that. I have walked into a building I have never been near in this life. I have no knowledge of this place, but I was able to visualize an event there, see the activities of people inside, know where the bathroom was, etc. I cannot explain how this could be. I believe that there are many forces and beings with this time and another time in the hemisphere. I believe in parallel universes. I am not sure if time is chronological, or if past times are gone, ended, or extend to the now. I will have knowledge that doesn't match my history. God is so vast in imagination and ability. Our ignorance of the entirety of the story is by His design. I grew up singing an old hymn, 'We Will Understand It Better, By and By.'"

One definition of a mystic is a person who accesses the invisible world. Barbara perceives Spirit through a felt presence, an altered sense of time, or an intuition. Barbara has eyes for thin places.

As we did with all of our couples, we asked Bobby and Barbara to reflect on their parents' deaths and the lessons taken away from them. As mentioned earlier, Bobby did not enjoy an emotionally demonstrative relationship with his father, yet in his story, we witness healing and loving at the end of life. As long as we take a breath, we can still grow, love, forgive, and heal.

Bobby began, "My father was a diabetic most of his life and died at the age of fifty-one from a stroke. I was twenty-three or twenty-four. Bedridden for the last four years of his life, he depended on someone to do everything. Estranged from him for many years, Mom took him in and provided care. I was stationed in the Air Force in DC and came home once a month to see him.

"I will never forget the particular day I visited my dad in the hospital. He seemed so old, but he was only forty-five or forty-six at the time. I fell on his bed and sobbed. We had a relationship where there was love, but we didn't show it. He struggled during the last six months. One thing I will take to my grave is the memory of when I came home the weekend before he died and brought my wife and kids. When we were getting ready to leave, he asked if we would come home the following week and bring Toni and young Bobby, my children. I said 'Yes,' but knew I wasn't coming. Friday, he died. Maybe he was waiting for me to bring my kids. It was sad, but we got through it."

Many of us look back on our relationships with our parents with love and regret. Bobby's love, compassion, and loyalty prevailed in his challenging relationship with his father.

Barbara also loved her father and disclosed the following story about his passing. "My father died in 2013. He'd never had a colonoscopy, and at age eighty-three, he sought medical care after experiencing sudden and profuse bleeding. He was diagnosed with colon cancer and died within several months. I talked to Daddy about his will, end-of-life decisions, and using heroic methods to maintain life. He said, 'If they've invented it, hook me up to it. Freeze me until there is a cure.' I asked, 'Are you serious?' and he was. Near the end, Daddy was hospitalized. I was in the room when the doctors said they were at the end of what they could do. He said, 'So Doc, is this it?' The doctor said, 'There are a couple of things we could do that could extend your life briefly, but your children will watch you reduce to nothingness.' I turned to him and said, 'So Daddy, you remember we talked about your last wishes?' He said, 'You tear that up. I don't want that.' I remember being so proud of him. He is my hero. Still is."

Barbara's relationship with her mother was more complex. "Conversely, my Mama and I weren't nearly as close. Something was missing in our relationship, so I always saw my grandmother as my real mother. She was easier to please and get along with, gentler and warmer. Mama had a stroke about thirteen years before her death. It affected her physically, but her mind was sharp. She was a tough old bird. I honor her toughness. Despite my tendency to be emotional and easygoing, I am proud that I can be tough, too, and stand up for myself when pushed.

"At eighty-four, Mama slipped when being transferred from her bed to a wheelchair, resulting in double fractures of the ankle of her one leg still capable of supporting her weight. The doctors did not recommend surgery. As complications mounted, my mom's leg was amputated to stop the spread of ensuing gangrene. Even after this drastic act, her health continued to decline. Not only did her organs begin to break down, but gangrene also found its way to her remaining leg. Like the rest of my family, I was in disbelief that Mama was nearing the end of her life. We would not put her through a second amputation, especially since her doctors told her it would only extend her life two to three months.

"I worried for my mama's soul. She was a very difficult woman in my mind, and in my judgment, she loved hearing bad news affecting other people. She loved and thrived on sadness and disappointment. She was mean-spirited. I had hoped her manner was the result of a mental illness and that she was not in control. Yet near the end, she dealt with a recurring issue she had before held against her only sibling."

Sharing more background, Barbara continued, "My mom became pregnant with me as a teen and was never confident in her relationship with my dad – even though the two were married before my birth. For about a third of the time in sixty-plus years, Mama estranged herself from her sister. She believed that when she was carrying me, her sister saw Daddy talking to another woman, but my aunt never told her. The issue was raised again – now, just before her death. Despite Mama's protestations that she never wanted to see her sister again, she told me upon my arrival for a visit that Ruth (my aunt) and hubby Ernie had just left. I immediately asked if she had been mean to them. Her response warmed my heart. She said, 'I decided it was time to stop my doubt and anger.' She renewed an important relationship days before her death."

Barbara and Bobby remind us that forgiveness and mercy are possible, even on our death beds and beyond. Many women carry "mother wounds," where their mothers were wounded from their own childhoods and lacked the capacity to provide love, safety, and warmth to their daughters. Attachment theories are better known and understood today. Barbara's story reminds us that our lives, while not Hollywood movies where everything neatly works out in the end, are capable of healing and grace in all conditions. When our parents die, many of us have to sort through intensely mixed feelings, regrets, grief, and gratitude and finally forgive reality for what it is. We sense these challenges are part of what makes us who we are.

Barbara concluded, "So much, I don't understand. When people are gone, you see their value in your life. I am older now. My siblings look at me as the matriarch, and when my time comes, if not suddenly, I hope to approach my demise much as my parents did. My dad died mouthing the words, 'How Great Thou Art,' as my family sang along. I can't imagine a better way to die."

While we only had three hours for this interview, you can see that we met them on the rich ground of story and truth. We will never forget being in the compassionate presence of Barbara and Bobby. As we concluded with our final question about their wisdom regarding relationships, aging, and living "side by side in Spirit," they noted how important love is.

When they were younger, Bobby and Barbara were busy moving on to the next thing, the next activity, or being right and winning arguments. With age, they highlight how they are wiser about relationships and what is truly important.

When they go to church holding hands, people express their surprise that they haven't been together forever.

"Love is important no matter how old you are, at any stage of life. Long gone is the assumption that only twenty-year-olds fall in love. You can love after losses, after a fiancé dies, after divorce, after a string of men who treated you poorly. There are good people you can rely on and love, no matter what your early experiences have been. That is it," were Barbara's final words to us. That is it.

To love is to make of one's heart a swinging door.

HOWARD THURMAN

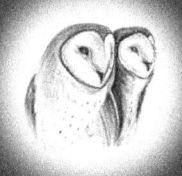

Blessed is the couple who
cares about the other's needs
as much as their own,
for they shall enjoy the
fruits of mutuality.

BLESSED IS THE COUPLE WHO

Enjoys the Fruits of Mutuality

INTRODUCING
SALLY HARE & JIM ROGERS

WHEN WE PULLED our RV into Jim and Sally's driveway in Surfside Beach, South Carolina, a handmade "Welcome Caryl & Jay" sign greeted us. Instantly at home, we proceeded to treasure a week filled with friendship, feasting, interviewing, and dog-walking by the sea a few blocks from their front door.

October is hurricane season, and we'd considered canceling our trip to the East Coast due to the dire forecasts, but thankfully did not. Upon arrival, we toured Jim and Sally's property and admired the recently installed sump pump designed to prevent flooding in the family room. Stepping over fallen branches from the last storm, we saw an Eastern box turtle peeking out from its shell to stare at us, and squirrels dashing over our heads across the tree branches. Under ongoing construction, the fairy garden contains a playful tribute to the nature spirits in their yard. Jim grieved aloud for the trees that came down in the last hurricane as the fence listed from the strong wind's impact.

Inside, sweet memorials line a wall with dog mugshots (Eleanor Roosevelt and Einstein, to mention two lost canine friends) of those who have passed over "the rainbow bridge." The photos stand as a testimony to Sally and Jim's commitment to rescuing dogs who have known human cruelty, been mistreated, abandoned, and otherwise unwanted. These dogs proceed to live very long, pampered lives in their care. Their current pooch, TBO, a gentle, black Goldendoodle gone deaf and almost blind, offers his friendly, calm presence to our nervous rescue dog, Lily Rose. Sally is a dog whisperer.

Jim and Sally met in the workplace. Both lived long, full, work-oriented lives before they met. Sally was the dean of graduate and continuing education at Coastal Carolina University and was considering becoming a college president (she changed her mind). Jim appeared one day looking for work in parenting and family life after a long and sometimes disappointing career as a producer, writer, and director of films in Charlotte, Atlanta, New York, and Los Angeles. Sally was not looking for a relationship and didn't want to get married. She was divorced in her twenties, whereas Jim was wed twice before. What stands out about their story are the ways they both vehemently eschewed the traditional roles that defined most marriages. Sally and Jim openly defied the traditional ways.

Sally reflected on her parents' relationship and her determination to avoid the same traps. "I grew up in Charleston, South Carolina, in the '50s, a time when gender roles were evident. My mother fell in love with my father at age ten and decided to marry him. As I grew up, they were very affectionate with each other, but I also witnessed that my father flirted a lot with other women and learned that this is what men did. Mom said that it doesn't matter because he always comes home. He had three daughters and wanted a son, and I became that. I grew up understanding love is not equal, and that the man's job was to make the woman feel safe, take care of her, then go out, work, and have a good time. But you stay together no matter what. I learned I wanted to be a man. When my first husband started acting like my father and having affairs, I divorced in my twenties. That was the beginning of my breaking out."

When Jim appeared at the university, she tried to fix him up with several women. Later, she would receive feedback from these women that all he wanted was to talk about her. And the talk about her entailed what he loved about her, which provided a mirror for how she wanted to see herself. They started dating.

Jim reflected on his family of origin history. "My family lived in a Norman Rockwell-like hometown in North Carolina. My father was a great provider, hardworking, honest, and full of integrity, and I hope I have taken that from him. My mother was the sweetheart, kind, gentle, and affectionate, and I got all of that too. But I didn't learn much about fathering; dad was emotionally detached. When he was sixty and dying of cancer, I asked him for a hug. I had never received a hug from my dad. I didn't know much about parenting except about being nice and kind. I got three spankings, and my parents never argued in front of us. My family cooperated, got along, and didn't fight.

"After the army, I tried to make my family into one like my parents'. But these were different times, and we had three children in diapers. How did that happen? It was tough, and I worked four jobs—as a TV station manager, an announcer for the weekend, on the production crews, and as a freelance writer on the side. I was not able to create a Norman Rockwell family. I moved up the ladder at work, traveled a lot, and that played havoc. I wanted to do better and differently, but I messed up."

If we were all so honest, most of us would feel compunction and sadness about our failures to live up to our ideals in our family lives.

Jim added, "People said to be forewarned when I was introduced to Sally, that she is a 'femiNazi,' with a reputation of being tough. My expectations for my life as an older person were not this. Holy crap, what is happening here? How did I, a country boy, end up with a Jewish girl with a PhD? I was supposed to be rich and famous by now, doing sitcoms. But it doesn't happen. I still wish I could have done that, but not to the point where I will pack my bags and move back to California."

Sally had to work through her judgments about Jim as well. "I thought he was too gentle, an older white man wanting work with parenting. But with his gentleness with family and his hugging, I came to understand it was maturity, a wintering into wisdom, and knowing that relationships are what matters, and are now his priority. He embodied wolf-ness and knew how to be with others. It was my misperception that he was too gentle. To say the least, my value of men was distorted. As I came to value his soft eyes and lovingness, I came to understand he didn't have to run with the wolves but to dance with them."

Sally continued, "I didn't want to marry again. I didn't want to have to ask permission from a husband. But Jim welcomed Mom, who lived with us during her last year of life. Our mutual agreement was to have her stay with us while she was dying of cancer. Watching Jim care for my mother with love and gentleness was how I knew he loved me. That is the kind of love he gives."

Sally realized that Jim saw her with "soft eyes," a spiritual notion of love that she learned in her travels. "Love is soft eyes.

When traveling for the Kellogg Fellowship in Bali, I learned that they see children as holy. They don't let their feet touch the ground for the first year of their lives. They would never mistreat a child. They would say, 'We see our children with soft eyes, not that we don't see sharp edges. Not that we don't see faults and shadows, but we see with soft eyes like there is Vaseline coating them. We see the faults and know that if the child lost those shadows, she would lose her gifts, and we wouldn't want to lose them. That is what we mean by soft eyes.'"

If love is an action verb, seeing each other in this manner is one practice Sally and Jim offer each other. They adore each other, create a safe and loving home together, and go out of their way to encourage and support one another in their many creative endeavors.

Sally highlighted another significant action Jim promised her as they were building trust. He proclaimed to her that he wanted to support her freedom to go, be, and do "who you are." Their love includes championing each other in each living up to their fullest potential. When Sally retired at age fifty-seven from the security and confines of her university career, they set up a business entitled still learning, inc. Sally has relied on Jim's encouragement and support as she traveled frequently and internationally, took risks, and created programs and retreats for many others, which entailed long periods away from Jim, who keeps the business end in order. He picks her up at the airport when she comes home and never complains about her schedule.

She concluded these reflections with, "As we age, it is harder and harder to leave home. Time is precious, and I realize this is where I want to be now." Now well into his mid-eighties, Jim's failing eyesight and advancing age are a growing concern. Jim is twelve years older than Sally. They want to be there for each other.

Jim said, "Sally is my third and last wife. I got married to my high school sweetheart when I was twenty. I didn't have a clue about what real love is, what responsibility is, or how to carry my role. It lasted nineteen years. My second one was different and more tormenting. There was no real love there. She wanted me to be a rich and famous director, and when it didn't happen, she was disappointed and turned to drugs and alcohol. When Sally and I met, this felt more like love, warmer and toastier. We grew so nicely into caring for and being with each other. I would rather be with her than anyone else. We hibernate. I am an inside person, content to stay in our nest and not socialize. I want to be with her. Sally didn't need me but liked me. This is a big difference, wanting to be with versus needing."

When Jim reached midlife, he sought ways to serve parents of young children, using his creative gifts for writing books, making films, teaching, facilitating parent education programs, and writing regular columns for several local papers. This work flavors their relationship. They don't understand how partners and parents can be so mean to each other and why they don't work harder on loving instead. Jim asks parents in his classes, "How can you say you love this child so much, yet you beat them?" They reply, "To get them to do what I want them to do," as if beating someone will bring about better behavior. His work is to teach different ways to influence children, but it is never an easy sell. Parents say things like, "I was spanked, and I turned out all right." We indeed follow our parents' examples unless we learn new ways.

Couples also make this mistake, emotionally beating each other up when disappointed rather than learning skills to help each other get what they need. Jim and Sally strive for mutuality in their relationship and to act in ways that say, "Your happiness is as important to me as my happiness."

Sally illustrated mutuality at play with a story. "My happiness is deeply entangled with Jim's happiness. Jim intensely listens to me. It is so amazing. Sometimes he knows what I want before I do. He listens in a way I have never known. For example, when we met, he was on his way to live in the mountains of North Carolina, where he feels a special kinship. I love living by the ocean. I have lived in this home by the sea for twenty-something years. We wondered, 'Do we sell?' We decided to add the log cabin he wanted to the brick beach house I already owned. This home became the intersection of Jim and Sally and how we live."

In the same manner in which they adore and nurture their adopted dogs, Sally and Jim have embraced the rigors and gifts of aging with courage, honesty, and humor. Sally leads retreats on this theme, while Jim has written books of poetry about aging and a play entitled *Geriatric Monologues*. It was elected for the Piccolo Spoleto Festival in Charleston.

Sally frequently proclaims, "I love being old." She likes the increased time and permission to go inward, not to worry about appearances, workplaces, and money, and the freedom to be as eccentric, wild, and outspoken as she wishes to be, which she does. Yet neither of them shies away from discussing the hardships of old age.

"Growing old is not a piece of cake," Jim noted. "I have good and bad days. I have written about how skin ages, droops, and sags. Parts of my body don't work as well, like my eyes, which are slowly going blind with macular degeneration. I can't hear so well. I have always been athletic, capable of blowing leaves off the roof and the heavy lifting that yard maintenance entails, but Sally insists I don't do something that stupid anymore. In terms of relationships, some intimacies are not the way they used to be. I keep saying to her that if she wants to travel to Europe again, go for it, but I am at the point I am not going to do that. I am glad I am going through aging with her. I try not to be as old as I am with Sally. She cooks and brings things to me when my legs don't work as well, getting up and down. I hate that and how it impacts our life together. But I am grateful to be with her." Jim is outspoken in his desire to eschew nursing homes and hospitals. And he realizes that anything can happen, any day.

An ongoing theme in Sally's work is connecting "soul and role." She now approaches aging with this intention in mind. "A touchstone of my life is the importance of noticing and naming what is changing in me and others as I connect soul and role with aging. Our culture does a terrible job with aging, but I don't want to get defensive and fight it, but notice. Many have noted there are more old people than ever but few elders. I am committed to finding new ways of naming getting older, then nurturing what I named in our relationship and the larger world. We are living longer, with more time after our careers, yet we are still not awake and aware of that, so we are squandering it. As a lifelong educator, who pays close attention to human development, anyone fifty-five and older is one age group in our culture. We aren't paying attention to the difference between the decades. When young children fall, we help them pick up and keep going. When older adults fall, it is a whole different thing. This stage of life is not a disease, but appropriate, normal development; we can notice, name it, and get better at what we can nurture."

Jim is candid about aging. "This is tough for me. I wish I could still eat anything I wanted and not worry about gaining weight. I wish I could conduct a two-hour class, moving around like I used to. Now I have to sit down. I get up, and it sounds like a wrestling match is going on . . . ooh, ooh, ahh, ah. I am all right, but I am old, and my body hurts. The acceptance is there, and I remind myself that at least I am not in a nursing home in a wheelchair, and I remember that I am fortunate. So I eat right, take meds, and eat fish. That is acceptance to me. Sometimes I do better than others."

Sally's natural optimism came through. "I want to co-create with my body, mind, and spirit as I age. I don't know what is possible, and I don't have good role models. As some things decrease, the potential for other things to increase is also there. I find this wintertime exciting."

Sally and Jim claim the importance of their sex lives and how they have to "figure it out." Sex matters to them. They enjoy sex as often as they can and claim it as the epitome of intimacy. Sally said, "For women, the idea of a sex life after menopause is new. We treat menopause like a disease, yet I barely knew I had gone through it. In Bali, only after menopause can women be considered equal to men. Before then, they are not allowed to serve as judges and in political offices. Learning about that has been important to me. Now, at this age, Jim has more estrogen than I do. I wish I could give him some of my testosterone. The gift of this age is that we laugh at this. Intimacy looks and feels different now. Our life is continuous foreplay."

Jim proclaimed that just touching each other is essential. No matter where they are, they are always touching and connecting. Sally concluded, "What I love about aging sex is the after play. In my experience with younger men, they went to sleep or went home. That just doesn't happen anymore."

In Jim's salty way, he added, "It is important to realize that everything doesn't break. Knees, etc., well, you have to keep working at it. I have deficient testosterone levels and can barely get out of my chair. So I get treatments when eight pellets of testosterone are injected into my butt. Afterward, I am a new person with lots of energy. Let's go dancing! At eighty-four, I ain't done yet."

According to Sally, "Spiritual and physical are in the same sentence." They articulate a sense of melting into each other, knowing this deep connectivity. "Our church is our time for loving each other. Jim has taught me the importance of touch, physical loving, kissing, and hugs. He taught my whole family how to hug. We want to give others the love we enjoy so that they might know this kind of love, reciprocity, and the gentleness of being in love."

Jim concluded, "With my first wife, if I didn't know she was sitting in the bedroom and I walked through from the bathroom naked, she would say, 'That is disgusting.' My second wife would say, 'I hope nobody sees you. I am so embarrassed. Why are you doing this?' But now, if I walk across the bedroom naked, Sally says, 'Oohhh, cute. You are so adorable.' You just don't get that from anybody." Aging with soft eyes.

Since Sally and Jim are both honest about the realities and opportunities of aging, we weren't surprised to find them equally open about facing death. Having experienced their parents' transitions from this life, they describe dying as a "thin place" and a central part of a spiritual process. While neither focuses on what happens after death, they did not shy away from discussing death and its mysteries.

Sally finds it "a great relief in knowing I won't live as long as I have lived. It is a real comfort to know that however much time remains, it is not seventy-two years! The uphill part is done. The downhill stage gives me a different kind of courage to know I am not here forever. I am more willing to take risks, be who I am, and to speak up because it is my only chance to do so. I have a responsibility to do that as an elder."

Sally's mother lived with them during her last year of life. "Being able to accompany my mother in the last nine months of her life was a great but painful gift. She had colon cancer that later metastasized. There was such learning in so many ways. The first part was about changing our roles as mother/daughter, not losing those roles, but now with me assuming many of the caregiver tasks. I struggled with how to do that in a way that didn't feel disrespectful. We couldn't fix her. This wasn't going to get better. A good death was the goal, but this time was not about getting well. In my first Circle of Trust program, Jim and my sister Jane experienced a clearness committee and were trained on how to ask open, honest questions and why we do not offer advice. The process invites the soul's wisdom from the person. At Mom's bedside, we felt like a clearness committee. We asked her open, honest questions, and there was so much learning for us. We couldn't fix her cancer, but we could offer her our presence and our listening. The circle's work also prepared me to have the courage to accompany someone dying without trying to fix them."[1]

Sally witnessed the "thin place" that the dying often experience. "The things Mom was able to see in the last months of her life, I couldn't see. She would say, 'Don't sit there. Your dad is sitting there. You will be surprised, but the Virgin Mary came to visit me. This is surprising because I am Jewish, but Mary was Jewish too. She brought a baby in, and that's what she does now. She welcomes babies.' At three or four in the morning, she was kicking under her covers, and when I asked her what she was doing, she said she was trying to open the window because there was a light on the other side. When I opened the window, she could see this beautiful light. I received these gifts and could share them with Jim because we were all living together."

When eldercare is "outsourced" or institutionalized, we sadly miss out on the mystical experiences common at the end of life. The dying speak metaphorically, like Sally's mom longing to open the window. She was ready to go into the Light and was looking for an opening. You honor them when you take them seriously.

Sally noted, "My father's death was different because Mom was still there and doing the caretaking. I felt the need to be there for her. I realized when she died, I was also grieving for my father because I hadn't done it at the time since I was caring for Mom during her loss. This is a reminder that there is always time for grieving, and there is no formula. With Jim's parents, I have gotten to know them through him, yet I know a sadness because I never met them in person."

"The story of Benjamin Button really speaks to me of how we can only understand life backward," Jim noted. "Dad died at sixty-one of pancreatic cancer, which he lived with for a year. He got down to ninety pounds. I was with him the day he died, and I remember it clearly. It was the only time I had a full-blown bawling cry at the back of the garage. I cried for two hours. We had never been close; we had the honoring of the father by the son but with little expression of affection.

"On the other hand, with my mother, I was in LA as she was declining in North Carolina. We don't understand the value of time with parents until we look back. One of my major regrets is thinking of my career and self, moving to LA, and wanting to be Mr. Hot-Shot film-maker, 3,000 miles across the country from where my mother was dying. We know we have to do this to be professionals in the world, but it is such bull. It is a violation of proper order. She was alone for two to three years and died of heart failure. That haunts me. I try to help my grandchildren understand that. These are tough memories."

In Jim's work with dysfunctional families, he notices that even when children were abused and never loved, when the parent dies, the grown child is heartbroken. Even in foster care, kids often want to go home, no matter how badly they were treated. The parent/child relationship is a profound connection, one we reflect upon our entire lives. Jim's regrets about not being emotionally close to his father in life, yet grieving deeply at his passing, is a repeated theme for the men in our interviews.

Jay often observes that many of his men friends carry a sense of "father hunger" or "father pain." Father hunger refers to missing their father's presence when growing up. The father's role was defined as "bringing home the bacon," which entailed disassociation from the family and shutting down their emotional and relational capacities. This pattern exemplifies the patriarchal model passed down through generations. Sometimes the "father pain" is a result of an unpleasant relationship with their fathers, where violence, drugs, alcohol, neglect, and emotional or physical abuse are involved. Fathers returning from Vietnam or other American conflicts, police jobs, etc., face even greater struggles with parenting. When the fathers die, acute grief at all that was lost—not just in death, but in life—can be overwhelming. We sincerely hope that this sad cycle of disconnection for men in this culture can end.

As our time together came to its natural conclusion and we unhooked our RV to prepare to continue our journey, Sally and Jim reminded us that "still learning" isn't just the name of their company but a way of life for them and a way of pursuing meaning.

In Jim's words, "If you don't have a sense of purpose, and get up and do something meaningful to you, life gets shorter and longer." He revealed his rage at how things are going in our country and how his voice as an elder is often ignored and marginalized. He is outraged at the lack of civility within our political system and the failure to create a just society that supports family life and economic equality. Sally affectionately reminded him of the reasons she wanted to hire him were his passion for parent education and for wanting a better world. She pointed out that within the word "rage" is the word "age." It is fair to say that Jim expresses the disappointment and compunction shared by the baby boomer generations in the winter of our lives. The high expectations and the idealism from "the Age of Aquarius" of our youth have indeed not been met, at least not in obvious ways. On the surface, things seem to be falling apart.

As Sally and Jim continue to offer their creative gifts to the world, their whirlwind of interests, ideas, and engagement creates a force field of beneficial presence. At the center of this dynamic energy is a peaceful, kind, loving relationship. Jim and Sally stand as examples of beneficial presence: abundant elder giving, elder sharing, elder loving, and elder wisdom.

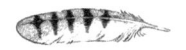

We have so many old people and so few elders.

CHARLES EISENSTEIN

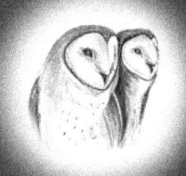

Blessed is the couple who
extends tender care to one another
when suffering, diminished,
wounded, or shamed,
for they shall be comforted.

BLESSED IS THE COUPLE WHO
Extends Tender Care When Suffering

INTRODUCING
ANNE & TOM BUTLER

DRAWING NEAR TO the Butlers' home, although a bit road-weary, we celebrated that we had made it across the entire country in our lumbering Winnebago and were excited to catch sight of a road sign in Greenville, South Carolina, pointing to a small town named Travelers Rest. Soon we would understand how the area got its name, a place for exhausted travelers herding their cattle from points north to Charleston, desiring a brief respite in their long journey. We could hardly wait to spend time with Anne and Tom.

Following the signs to Paris Mountain, our RV slowly began the 2,000-foot ascent. Within a half-mile, we were at their front door. We instantly experienced their mountain home as *a sanctuary of care*, where, like Laurie and Gary, they extend the gift of spiritual hospitality.

A vista viewed from their back deck takes in a vast landscape that establishes a peaceful sense of spaciousness. Tom, a photographer, mentioned the tranquil beauty of winter sunrises that light up dissipating cloud formations in the skyscape. Their guest room offers a special place for friends and sojourners not only to lay down their bags but, for some, also to lay down their heavy burdens. It reflects a simple but elegant beauty equipped with tea, coffee, a small refrigerator, fresh flowers, soft pillows, warm blankets, a relaxing chair on the balcony, and seasonal images of places they have traveled together. Year-round, the Butlers' inviting guest room is frequently occupied by friends on retreat from the fray of their lives.

In our initial conversation, we learned that Anne and Tom enjoy living only ten minutes away from Furman University, a charming campus with a large lake at its center. The lake's perimeter is about one-and-a-half miles, and during their many lake walks—one season following another—they savor and share many soulful conversations. "Walking is a contemplative practice for us," Anne said, "Our frequent walks have become a 'cadence of grace' wherein we listen to each other with the ears of our hearts."

Being in their presence, we also entered a cadence of grace. You know you are in the company of caring souls when they make you feel like the most important person in their lives, which is how we felt with Anne and Tom. We were reminded of how the Irish monasteries served pilgrims in ancient times. Travelers were always welcome to stop, rest, enjoy a meal, solicit spiritual support, and receive a blessing as sustenance for the road ahead.

On our first sun-filled morning together, camera rolling, we asked Anne and Tom the question, "What brought you together?" The Butlers' account of falling in love reflects the myriad ways couples find each other and commit to a life together. Stories become sacred stories when they reveal how every challenge, limitation, failure, gift, and talent is transformed into a genuine good when people not only survive but flourish.

Before marrying, Tom and Anne had similar backgrounds that ultimately brought them together. Both entered religious communities focused on serving God in the poorest of the poor, founded by a 16th-century French Saint, Vincent de Paul. Tom became a priest within the Congregation of the Mission (the official name for the men's community). Anne was a religious sister within the Daughters of Charity for seventeen years.

Tom spent most of his ministerial life in education and spiritual retreat leadership. He recalled, "I remembered her as Sister Anne McCleary. I met her many years ago as a priest, having given several retreats to the Daughters of Charity." In the years since they met, Anne had left her religious order, finding new ways to serve as a nurse practitioner, healthcare consultant, grief counselor, servant leader, and end-of-life doula. It was a combination of her new roles and what Tom remembered about Anne's character that led him to reach out in a time of need.

"I was deeply struck by her instinctive honesty, transparency, and gentle spirit. She was then and is today, a woman whose beauty is soul deep. Her blue eyes pierce through you with a message that conveys a desire to see you, hear you, to know and be known by her. Her authenticity and spontaneous care are self-evident.

"I was not surprised to find such a supportive and compassionate response to my need. My need? I needed help with my brother, Richard, who had developed metastatic bladder cancer. He lived alone, and I needed guidance on the best ways to care for him so he could live well until he died. Anne graciously offered to come to Philadelphia from Baltimore to meet with my brother and be of service to both of us."

Tom admires one of Anne's hallmarks, her capacity to tend to the sick and dying with care and reverence. "She views each patient as a person blessed in their brokenness and beautiful in their vulnerability. Each encounter is treated as holy, where love is the best slow medicine, and death is not a disease to be cured but rather a sacred threshold infused with profound ache and awe.

"In this bittersweet encounter with Anne, I (we) fell in love. I often refer to this experience as my Abraham moment. In the book of Genesis 12:1, God tells Abraham, 'Go from your country and your father's household to the land I will show you.' I felt called to leave everything I knew and surrender to what I believe God was inviting us into together, side by side and heart to heart. I eventually processed my request for a dispensation from my vows as a priest through the Vatican. Today, with Anne, we continue to walk by faith and in abiding love."

The Pope ultimately granted Tom's dispensation after they had followed the two years of prescriptive guidelines dictated by the Church to have their marriage blessed, a requirement that was of vital importance for Anne's mother's peace of mind. Her mother, a devout and ultra-conservative Catholic, felt deeply torn that her daughter would marry a priest.

Anne said, "The hardest losses in my life have been the places where I expected love and it wasn't there." She related the profound sadness she carries in her memory from their wedding day. Anne believed in her heart that her mother would attend her wedding. As they walked into the small chapel, waiting hand-in-hand to walk down the aisle together, Anne's eyes scanned the small group of gathered friends looking for her parents. They were not there. Her eyes welled with tears as she squeezed Tom's hand even tighter. Somehow, she knew this was only the beginning of tending painful feelings of grief, betrayal, and emotional abandonment.

Anne and Tom believe it was no coincidence that their wedding day, September 14, 2001, had been named by President Bush as a national day of mourning following the horrific tragedy three days earlier of 9/11. The universal became the personal as her apprenticeship with sorrow unfolded before their eyes in their paradoxical dance of deep love and profound grief.

Anne disclosed that her faith is not defined by institutional dogmas and doctrines but rather by the heart and soul of authentic, loving, messy, life-giving relationships. Such was the crucible of human love they desired to live into with each other *and* with her parents. "With the tincture of time, and countless acts of loving-kindness, seen and unseen, my mother began to befriend Tom," Anne said. "He loved her unconditionally and wholeheartedly. He would do anything for her. On her terms and in her own time, she loved him in noteworthy and beautiful ways. I hold great peace that we were able to find a place in our hearts for forgiveness before she died. I believe today, she sees things very differently. And that is holy!"

Anne mentioned a special moment one month after her mother died. Her mother worked for the Daughters of Charity in Emmitsburg as a docent at the Shrine of St. Elizabeth Ann Seton for many years. In her memory, the Sisters who deeply loved and admired her wanted to have a memorial Mass celebrated at the Shrine. Anne recalled, "Tom asked me if I was going to speak about my mother at the liturgy. He thought it would be a wonderful opportunity to offer a reflection that was true and revealed the love we shared despite much heartache. I told Tom that my mother never thought it was proper for women to be in the sanctuary or participate in the liturgy, and I did not want to disregard this value that she held in life now that she had died. Tom responded, 'She is looking at you now with a whole different gaze.' Tom assured me he would be there with me. It was such a healing moment to speak about my mom, give thanks, celebrate, and remember the many moments of love that we shared on earth. I believe she now experiences this all in full measure and flowing over in heaven."

The absence of Anne's parents at their wedding placed Tom in a unique position to care for Anne as she suffered the trauma that ensued. In the interviews and in our own relationship, we have witnessed that partners helping each other with their family-of-origin issues is one of the greatest gifts couples offer one another. Tom's instinct to invite Anne into a new understanding of her mom was in service to her soul.

The interview question "What brought you together?" initiated the sharing of many stories where risk and change, vulnerability and courage, walk side-by-side with the Butlers. The following story humorously reflects this reality. Before they married, Tom came to Anne's apartment for dinner one night. Anne told him that they needed to put something on their wedding rings. Tom paused and looked reflectively up at the ceiling and then said, "How about love changes everything?" Anne stared at him, almost incredulous at his response. Then, collecting herself, she said, "I mean MONEY! We need to put money on our rings. They are on layaway, remember?" They could not stop laughing as they recounted this story. Tom heartily agrees that Anne is the pragmatist in the relationship, and he is the poet.

Our next question for them was, "What has most tested your love?" Tom, coming from a family where his father was an alcoholic, recognized how his childhood engendered a sense of shame and low self-esteem. This disposition gave rise to a pleaser personality that seriously impacted his physical, mental, and spiritual health. He noted that when his self-esteem wanes, their conflicts tend to be significantly higher. This is a predominant theme in Tom's life that he has spent much time addressing in counseling.

In Anne's family, dealing with emotions and conflict was never encouraged. "I grew up in a family with little room to express anger, frustration, hurt, and sadness. We were told to offer it up to God, or the feelings were not recognized, which implied they were insignificant. Tom's experience with the effects of his father's debilitating alcoholism on him and his family allowed little room to address conflict. Our religious formation did not afford us the pathway of addressing these issues; they too mirrored a similar pattern as found in my family system, encouraging us to pray more and look for a greater good."

So how do individuals address these challenging family patterns, much less integrate their meaning as a couple? As Anne described, there is no quick fix but a process that unfolds with time and intention.

"I began my apprenticeship with sorrow throughout many years of accompanying the sick and the dying, witnessing their courage and vulnerability. Through their suffering, I discovered a crucible for my transformation, which deepened my desire to become ever more real, forgiving, and loving in my life and marriage. I engaged in counseling and found it a tremendous blessing that encouraged me to befriend these parts of me and view them as vital messengers in my healing and wholeness. These wounds left unrecognized and untended can make or break any relationship. Often, what I leave unspoken out of fear of discord becomes a breeding ground for greater sorrow and emotional disengagement from myself and others. I pray with Richard Rohr's insight—pain that is not transformed is transmitted. I don't want to be a transmitter of pain but rather a bridge builder and instrument of healing."

Richard Rohr also opines that spiritual transformation comes from great love and great suffering. Committed relationships are intimately linked with our spiritual formation because they often mirror our inner wounds and the places we need healing. Anne and Tom's love is seldom far from their experience of great suffering.

The Celtic notion of the *Anam Cara* (soul friend) embodies the wisdom to "lean into the pain," highlighting the paradox that emotional pain worsens when we avoid it. Anam Cara captures the energy signature of Anne and Tom. They eschew the trap of "spiritual bypassing" their human problems and inner darkness by humbly facing them. To "lean into the pain" when experiencing conflict—when each person can quickly regress into fight-or-flight instincts—often entails calming down, witnessing the reactivity within, and choosing to mindfully respond, versus reacting.

As we explored their relationship with conflict, they pointed to two magnetic plaques prominently displayed on their refrigerator. Anne bought one at a shop in a small Vermont town that reflects her practical nature: "Don't go to bed angry. Stay up and fight." She jokingly told Tom this was her marriage motto. Feeling up to the challenge, the poet in him responded a few days later with a plaque of his own that he placed underneath hers that read, "Peace Prayer of St. Francis—Lord, make me an instrument of your peace." Like their "ring" story, the pragmatist and the poet have their share of conflicts. Anne sees conflict as an opportunity for greater engagement and emotional intimacy.

Tom stated, "I ask, 'How can we use a lens that invites Spirit into this conflict?' I have found that answer is the difference between reacting and responding. If I take time and pause before responding to the situation, I have already stepped into Spirit. Then, by inviting my truer self to respond, I uncover the spiritual response. 'How do I respond with kindness, compassion, and understanding?' is another question I ask. These questions draw upon my invitational, spiritual capacities versus instinctive, impulsive reactions in self-protection, anger, or revenge. I would sum it up by highlighting that *responding versus reacting* is a way of inviting in Spirit. I have to be humbly open in a conflict to the reality that I could be responsible for it. Am I open enough, vulnerable enough, to own that? Just asking this question has the power to defuse tension. Is it my fault? I am sorry."

When we asked "What has most challenged your love?" Anne recalled when she was days away from graduating with a master's degree in nursing from Catholic University in Washington DC in 2007. She was also working full-time as director of palliative care at Holy Cross Hospital. Tom's heart disease was becoming more pronounced, along with his symptom burden. She felt a gnawing wonder about her life's purpose and where she was being led at this threshold of her life.

In this moment of anguish on her last day of formal classes on campus, she recalled a patient she assisted during his extended hospitalization in the ICU. His simple manner, spiritual heart, and wisdom came to her as a quiet voice inviting her to connect with him. Anne remembered he was a car mechanic who owned a small garage only minutes away from the university campus, so she went there. Amid his disheveled garage, the elderly Jamaican man recognized her immediately. Seeing him again, she began to cry. He said, "My dear, sit here." He opened his desk drawer and pulled out an old, worn, tattered Bible. He invited Anne to put her hand on the Bible and close her eyes. He gently began to sing to her, "God will take care of you. God will take care of you." The rhythmic refrain echoed in her heart. His song transported her to an entirely different place. To this day, whenever she is struggling, Anne continues to hear his voice and words of reassurance, "God will take care of you." She knows she is not alone.

Anne believes that what disturbs us is what eventually nourishes us. Tom was diagnosed with coronary artery disease in August of 2009. In June of 2017, he needed to undergo open-heart surgery. Anne has endured her share of ambulance trips to the ER, hours in waiting rooms, endless nights of Tom's waxing and waning symptoms, and long periods of uncertainty. Good health is not promised to anyone. Anne and Tom face this unrelenting reality in their marriage by cultivating a healthy reliance on Spirit. They greet Tom's heart disease with a commitment to do what they can to stay healthy and live each day as if it were their last. This nourishes their awareness of what possibilities are within their grasp by believing that good can come from this heartache. And it has.

Anne and Tom's wall plaque in their "sanctuary of care" captures the idea that enlivens their way of the heart. *In the end, what matters most is, how well did you live, how well did you love, and how well did you learn to let go.* They have an intuitive sense of living their lives from the inside out and encouraging others to do the same. The home that Tom and Anne co-create as a sanctuary is also a base camp for learning and evolving. Anthropologist Mary Catherine Bateson (daughter of Margaret Mead and Gregory Bateson) once told Krista Tippett during an *On Being* interview how research affirms that the distinguishing quality of humans is a unique capacity for learning throughout the lifecycle.[1] Humans are constantly creating, changing, playing, and improvising as artists of our own lives.

For example, Anne and Tom initiated a practice based on John O'Donohue's poem "At the End of the Day: A Mirror of Questions" found in his book *To Bless the Space Between Us*.[2] In this reflective litany, O'Donohue suggests twenty-two questions that anyone can use to encourage greater self-awareness and emotional intimacy. Anne and Tom choose three or four questions in the evening to invite a deeper sharing and review of the day. This practice keeps them current, aware, and honest. Simple questions like "How are you within?" can open beautiful conversations, just waiting to be engaged.

Anne notes how the questions evoke some of the inner truths of the day just lived. Without an invitation, the subtle, uncomfortable feelings remain hidden. These questions enable them to connect on a soul level. Here they can keep a reality check on what is happening both within them and in the world around them.

Our final question was, "What do you hope your legacy will be as a couple?" Anne said, "The questions I do not ask myself, I won't ask Tom. To the degree I am willing to cultivate a courageous and generous spirit to see myself in my shadow and light, as God sees me, then I bring beauty, vulnerability, and truth to my marriage. If I refuse to do this, I compromise my growth and Tom's growth. After Tom's open-heart surgery, a friend asked if he could see Tom's scars. This stands as a powerful metaphor for me. When we can gently reveal and gaze at our own and each other's scars (seen and unseen) with compassion and tender love, they are softened and become pathways of healing and renewal."

Tom continued, "The legacy I wish to leave as a couple is that Anne and I were truth-tellers. That we were a married couple so committed that we ran the risk of being completely honest. In that honesty and vulnerability, we became even more alive. Real and loveable like *The Velveteen Rabbit*, a story we both love. This is a work in progress, but I have come to believe is vitally necessary if any relationship is to endure and, more importantly, flourish."

One final grace note comes from Tom's experience at the time of his father's death. We use it to close this chapter because it reflects for all of us in relationships how we must hold, in our hearts, both the ache and the awe at the core of most relationships.

"At age fifty-two, my father was diagnosed with a cancerous tumor located in the center and behind his lower jaw. As a firefighter, he took in more smoke than was healthy; as a cigarette smoker (Camels, no filter), he pushed the odds of getting cancer exponentially. As a drinker, well, he hit the trifecta of cancerous-causing agents. Debilitating surgeries left him with the whole lower part of his face removed and eighty percent of his tongue also taken away. Plastic surgeons did a remarkable job of trying to rebuild his face, yet there was no mistaking his painful scars and the fact he could not eat or speak. He lived for thirteen years with this disability.

"One day after a bad cold, probably pneumonia, his heart stopped, and we got him to the ER, but the likelihood of his survival was hours, not days. When he died in the emergency room, I stood with my mother as she came to look in on him for the last time. With tears streaming down her face, she took her hand and ran it over his scarred face saying: 'Oh, my beautiful husband.' I froze the frame at that moment and have never forgotten the scene or her words. It is with me today as if it happened yesterday. My deepest desire for Annie and me is that we will always be able to see the beauty in one another, despite our sicknesses, aging, failures, dementia, or disability. It is also my hope for all couples. My mother's example of unconditional love inspires me to love Annie wholeheartedly. I will always be grateful for her witness."

At the end of our days, when holding each other's hands, we can all pray for this grace: that we will have lived our relationship in such a way that we can cherish each other, seeing past trauma-laden human scars and wounds to the deeper essence of our souls, with the perspective of eternity.

Love is our true destiny. We do not find the meaning of life by ourselves alone—we find it with another.

THOMAS MERTON

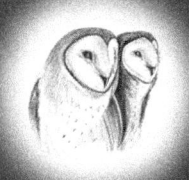

Blessed is the couple who
recognizes the Indwelling Spirit
in all of life, for they shall
encounter the Mystery and
see the Light in all beings.

BLESSED IS THE COUPLE WHO
Recognizes the Indwelling Spirit in All of Life

INTRODUCING
PATSY GRACE & HARVEY BOTTELSEN

WHEN WE FIRST entered the home of Patsy and Harvey in the hills above Santa Barbara, California, we couldn't take our eyes off of what surrounded them in the living room: various pillar crystals in many different shapes and sizes, sometimes a foot or taller, collected from their world travels. Instantly we realized the unseen world has a tangible presence here. Jay and I have collected a few crystals ourselves over the years. Crystals are considered "master healers" of the mineral world that amplify and regulate energy. They are also known for aiding concentration and memory. Since concentration is a crucial dimension of intelligence, we realized we were in for an exciting interview and rare encounter. We weren't disappointed as we explored their story of coming together and staying together. Patsy and Harvey embody a unique capacity for awareness and many perspectives.

Although both were living in Southern California at the time, Patsy and Harvey met in Bali, Indonesia, an island well known for its sacred sites and beauty. When touring the ancient Elephant Cave, their eyes met, and they experienced a powerful transfer of energy and information that they claim to still not entirely understand. Patsy and Harvey now name this intense connection as divinely orchestrated, as destiny, and as an initiation. They spotted something in the other that held a charge, a deep recognition, and resonance, what some might call a soul mate.

If you believe in synchronicity and the power of beginnings, you may be curious about the cave where they met. The Elephant Cave served as a sanctuary and bathing site dating from the 11th century. It contains both Hindu and Buddhist imagery, including a *lingam* and *yoni* and the image of Ganesh, the Hindu god with the head of an elephant. The cave itself was discovered in 1923, but the fountains and bath were discovered in 1954.

In Hinduism, *yoni* is Sanskrit for "source," "womb," or "vagina." It is the feminine symbol of the Goddess Shakti, the consort of Shiva. The yoni is often associated with the lingam, a short, phallic, cylindrical pillar-like symbol of Shiva, usually made from stone, metal, gems, wood, or clay. Shiva represents the generative power of existence, all creativity, and fertility at every cosmic level.

Patsy and Harvey, reflecting on their initial meeting, considered why they were brought together so intensely. Friends tell them that they are a model of a good relationship, which is hard for them to grasp. Patsy believes their "mission" as a couple is to explore how to balance masculine and feminine qualities within themselves and with each other. Throughout their marriage, they have pursued meditation and a spiritual path together and continue to explore the changes around us in this culture as gender fluidity becomes an acceptable topic of conversation. Integrating feminine and masculine principles within us is a high value and key to the evolution occurring in humans today.

In Harvey's words, "We are learning to live in the paradox of it all. A paradox, not this or that but both/and thinking and being. This culture has such an either/or dualistic mindset in terms of gender identities. Now, what is happening in terms of man/woman identity is changing. For instance, on Facebook, there are seventy-plus gender identities one can claim. Things are changing in terms of what it is to be male and female, which is incomprehensible for many of us older folks. In our time, boys were boys and girls were girls. Younger people get it. They have permission to live out of this box. This is just one example of the mystery unfolding in our world."

This loosening of rigid gender roles that defined the patriarchal patterns in our generation's relationships is an emergent pattern, and Patsy and Harvey actively embrace this change. They are a couple who are genuine explorers, adventurous spiritual pilgrims at heart, as their beginnings suggest.

Three years into their relationship, they were introduced to an international spiritual teacher and channel known as Lazaris, whose teachings grew to become a central organizing principle of their relationship. Patsy explained, "Since then, that has been most of what we have done in terms of activities. We also created a spiritual family, now our closest friends, who come together to hear this teacher. It is so embedded in our lives, and what we do every day, that it is kind of hard to describe. Because we have embodied it so much, it is a part of our beingness. How do you breathe? You just do it."

Harvey continued, "It is a relationship with all that is, including the dark experiences. It is not a church or worship, but an ongoing progression of beingness with all that is."

Their practices include daily meditation, talking together about their experiences and looking for the meaning in them, and relating them to the bigger picture and the implications for humanity. From their study with Lazaris, Patsy named a quality that permeates their experience. "Both of us have a desire and goal of living an enchanted life. Because of that, we see enchantment everywhere. They are the highlights that happen daily. We are on a kind of plateau because as you become sensitive to beauty, creativity, and love, enchantment is everywhere; it is tuning in to a higher vibrational level. This is more a way of being. It is always, everywhere with us."

Harvey added, "The word 'enchantment speaks' to the nature of reality. Evolution has been about impact, causation, things pushed around, striving, making commitments, and achieving. That type of reality is reaching its limits in terms of being the only way to live. The consciousness behind our actions is what matters. What is the intention behind that behavior? This paradigm is based on how we think about the nature of reality."

He continued, "Back in the day, for the indigenous people, everything was enchanted. Scientists are now starting to talk about enchantment again. With two electrons, you can send one off, then manipulate one, and the other responds. That is more the accurate and mystical nature of reality. We work hard to demystify this and put it into our language. Language emphasizes nouns. As we move into more of an inner life, the sense of beingness is more important. Great traditions begin with the 'beingness' experience which has innate attunement with beauty and joy; it is just being present. You can experience that. It has great power. We are describing the way we have found to do that."

Patsy added, "I think that if one looks at spirituality as your relationship with God, or the Goddess, or All That Is, then that means you move into a place where you see yourself in relationship with everything: people, trees, land, air. Everything has an impact on you, and you have impact on everything else. When you can hold that, your life does become enchanted, not just in your small world, but in the big world. Everything is alive, breathing, interacting, and moving together. Everything is mystical. One of my mottos, which I use a lot, is 'I surrender my separateness.' It is often challenging, especially when someone is off-putting to me, but it is an interesting exercise. This is where we need to go, to realize there is a Oneness and we are a part of it."

So many thought leaders, in the face of our many challenges globally, are calling for this kind of unity consciousness, claiming that if we don't start living as though we are related, humans will destroy themselves. Sitting with Patsy and Harvey, we felt blessed with their practical, place-based, enchanting wisdom.

Richard Rohr has named this "enchantment" consciousness the "Universal Christ,"[1] which redefines incarnation, traditionally used in reference to Jesus. Nowadays, this phrase refers to the spirituality in all matter and the resulting sense of the profound interconnectedness of creation. Harvey and Patsy have dedicated their lives to this shift towards experiencing the web of interconnectedness as the ground from which human beings create a different future. Until a new consciousness is achieved, nothing can change. They believe our survival depends on enchantment.

Yet like all couples, Harvey and Patsy also live in their bodies and very human natures. After their initial enchanting connection in the Elephant Cave, they encountered their differences. Both students of the Enneagram, Harvey is a type Three, while Patsy is a type Eight. They acknowledge that these two types are not easily cohesive. As an Eight, Patsy is a feeling body type, for Eights experience life as an intense emotional body blow, and freely express their anger. In contrast, Harvey is a deep thinker who tends to live in a world of ideas.

When we asked Patsy for an example of how she works with their issues, she noted, "What has helped us both is our commitment to our growth, to looking at ourselves, and learning to love each other but ourselves as well. For example, not long ago, I found myself in an old loop. I was upset with Harvey, and when upset, I often withdraw. I removed myself physically from the situation, and what popped into my head was that when I react this way, I am hurting myself. I am not respecting myself enough to say, 'Hey, what is going on? We have to address this.' A switch went off. I can't do that anymore. It is not respecting myself, our relationship, and it is not moving us forward."

Harvey added, "Learning how to act with respect has been a growing edge. We must be willing to go deep enough into our differences to respect them and learn from them. We need to learn to sense what the other is feeling. It can take you to a place you wouldn't be going alone. I am learning to respect all of that, rather than just go to judgment."

When we asked, "What has most challenged your relationship?" they revealed an incident that is still difficult for them to revisit. When they met, Patsy ran her own company in LA, and Harvey worked in businesses in Santa Barbara and LA. Putting together their lives, including children from Harvey's first marriage, was not always easy. Five years into their relationship, Harvey heard a loud voice in his head claiming he needed to live by himself for a while, and he subsequently asked Patsy to move out. As a result, they separated.

In Harvey's words, "This was a poignant moment. I saw its impact on Patsy, and I just wanted to jump off a cliff that I had hurt her so much. This was before we were married."

Patsy added, "But I now think it was necessary. When we met, I was still living in LA, had a business, and went back and forth. We lived in different cities and were not together every day. When I moved in, Harvey was not ready for it, and shortly after, both of his adult children moved back home too. I had been single my whole life and was in my late 40s. I was used to having my own business, my own life. Suddenly I was here, and everyone else came back. Harvey was shaken. We lived like that for a couple of years until he told me to leave. I had divested myself of my old life in LA. It broke me when he said that. It took us some time to get through it, but now I see it was necessary."

Harvey said, "Nothing changes until you do. When I point my finger at someone, three fingers point back at me. This is a truism of life and in our relationship. It is necessary to do your work, for your relationship can't grow and expand unless you do."

As Patsy and Harvey reflect on aging and growing older, they both celebrate the freedom and softening it offers from the intensity of careers and managing businesses. They now prioritize their spiritual lives, have taken the time to travel extensively, and give back. They are aware of the value of extending their presence in all of their encounters and strive to approach life with a gentler softness.

Harvey has encountered some arduous health challenges, whereas Patsy, younger by about seven years, has not, except for menopause. Harvey noted that men don't generally feel their aging until they hit their seventies, and as the other men in these interviews reveal, it is tough on one's identity. Being athletic all of his life, a tennis pro and eventual owner of the Santa Barbara Tennis Club, he recently had to quit the game after an accumulation of bodily injuries, including two hip replacements. In 2011 he went in for a check-up and underwent heart bypass surgery. He notices that his short-term memory is beginning to waffle a bit.

When we wondered how these physical challenges impacted their relationship, Harvey said, "I depended on Patsy so much when an infection attacked and settled in my spine's T3 and T4 areas, which was quite serious. The doctors were perplexed. She was giving me daily injections of antibiotics for three months. It was a matter of surrendering to where I was. But it was challenging being with this and the fear factor; I wondered, 'Is this going to get better?' Hospitals lose most patients with these infections. I was facing my transition."

In this season of life, a health problem can change everything. Whether it arrives suddenly, or gradually, all couples undergo these changes. "When Harvey had his heart issue, it was unexpected," Patty related. "He went in for an angiogram, and the doctor came out and told me his heart was 98 percent blocked. He said to me, 'We call this the widow maker.' They scheduled him to have triple bypass surgery by 2 p.m. that afternoon. I thought, 'What? He was playing tennis the day before.' My response was to step into the champion role of the Enneagram type Eight and protect him. I sent emails to everyone, saying this is happening, send prayers, but don't come or call. Send me a text. I kept people advised.

"He was in the hospital for only two days, and they sent him home. It was shocking. They didn't tell me anything about how to care for him. I allowed no visitors until he could sit in a chair and talk. I became Mama Bear and kept everyone away. We spent six weeks this way, just the two of us. I was also careful to care for myself."

Looking back on this time, Harvey calls Patsy his "superhero." Reflecting on his years focused on sports, he now wonders if he still had the body of a twenty-year-old, would he do it again? From the wisdom and perspective of his age, he is not so sure it would be such a high priority and can now see the cost it exacted.

Neither of them shied away from discussing death. The Bower Foundation, where Harvey has served as board chair since its inception, has created opportunities in Santa Barbara for people to discuss death, explore many dimensions of end-of-life care, and how to improve the quality of life as we transition from this life. The goal of this work is both simple and radical: to decrease the fear of death in Santa Barbara.

Together, Harvey and Patsy participated in a small group program where they wrote and discussed their "Five Wishes," a program for advanced-care planning which outlines end-of-life preferences and plans.[2] When the Bower Foundation began funding this work over ten years ago, it was countercultural and revolutionary. Supporting the coordination of hospices and hospitals and other caregivers in the community through the formation of the Alliance for Living and Dying Well, these efforts continue to impact change in how the dying are cared for in Santa Barbara.

Many people wonder how to find meaning and life purpose as they age. We found this couple deeply engaged in meaningful spiritual practices, raising consciousness, and giving back. Stephen Cope writes about the nature of dharma and how it is born mysteriously out of the intersection between our gifts and the times in which we live. Dharma is a response to the urgent need of the moment, in the little corner of the world that is ours to transform.[3]

In our times, and in his corner of the world, Harvey discussed how he is working on a film and book project to portray his vision of what we are collectively experiencing as a spiritual paradigm shift during massive challenges.

"I am focusing my time on creating the New Paradigm Project. I have been thinking about this for a long time, looking at the big picture of the evolution of humankind. Consciousness, where we have been, where we are going—I can see there is a direction when I see the map. This is very stimulating for me to make a difference in the world. There is something extraordinary going on right now, and change is accelerating quickly, which looks like apparent chaos fed through the news media. But as I see it, some wonderful things are going on, and that is what I am committed to."

Patsy finds herself eschewing a focus on "doing" and embracing life as one with many opportunities to pursue her passions and time with family. "It is pretty opposite from Harvey in that I have a lot of passions, things I like to do, and interests. I don't feel there is something for me to 'do' in the world, or if there is, it is not clear right now. My passion is allowing that and not trying to do some things I know aren't right for me, which is challenging in this world. We are still in the model of 'doing is achieving.'"

Patsy extends loving attention to her large extended family and her wise presence to her friends. Many elders thrive in this way. When asked about maturity, she returns to her core practice in life, living from a place of enchantment and connection to Spirit. "Real maturity goes back to the Oneness; the wise person understands they are a piece of the Oneness, unique, and a critical piece of the One. That awareness is a part of maturity, a way of stepping into wisdom."

As we concluded the interview, we asked Harvey and Patsy what they hope their legacy will be, and they didn't hesitate to name something to which many parents aspire—unconditional acceptance of their children. Both Patsy and Harvey have led large lives, explored the far reaches of consciousness and spirituality, traveled the world, owned businesses, and contributed to the community of Santa Barbara significantly. Yet they didn't mention any of this. What they named was showing support for the next generation—their children, nieces, nephews, and grandchildren.

"I guess for me if I had a hope, it would be that my kids were able to see me the way I was, with all the facets of a father with a limited perspective on things, who was challenging for them, but also understand how I grew and was a value in their lives," Harvey said. "That I matured in the capacity to love them and they felt loved is important to me. I want them to say, 'My father accepted me, loved me, just the way I am.' This is a work in progress, and I know they have baggage from how critical I was of them when they were growing up. I still judge, but at least I know that judgment separates and hurts. To the extent I can accept my children just the way they are is huge. They can feel it if I do not. But if I can get to a place where I can do that, it frees them and frees me."

Patsy, who did not have her own children, continues, "I guess it is different for me because I am not their parent, so I am in a better position. They haven't lived with me 24/7 for many years. I want them to know they were loved, that I would always be there for them, and they would sense that having me in their life changed their life to a certain extent."

In his book *Living Your Unlived Life*, author Robert Johnson offers a powerful insight about parenting:

> Swiss psychiatrist Carl Jung wrote that 'the greatest burden a child must bear is the unlived life of the parents,' by which he meant that where and

> how our parents were stuck in their development or failed to follow their passions becomes an internal paradigm for the child also to become stuck. Frequently we find ourselves dealing with a parent's unresolved issues. At times we may replicate the patterns of our ancestors, or we may rebel and attempt to do the opposite. Interestingly, antagonism to the influences of parents binds just as tightly as compliance. Perhaps this fact is behind the ancient biblical admonition that the sins of a man shall be visited 'upon the children's children, unto the third and to the fourth generation.'"[4]

Harvey's comments on legacy reflect his commitment to acknowledge the places where he believes he fell short in his caring for his children by being too judgmental (what parent doesn't feel that way?) and his attempts to change. What a gift to the next generation.

We can't help but celebrate this couple for their candor and their enchanted, humble, beautiful presence in the world.

Enchantment is the belief that everything in nature is alive, wondrous, conscious, and a connected part of Consciousness and expressions of One.

LAZARIS

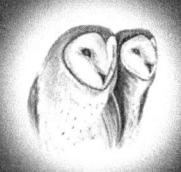

Blessed is the couple who
dances with the tension
between "me" and "we,"
for they shall know companioning
without loss of self.

BLESSED IS THE COUPLE WHO
Dances with the Tension Between "Me" & "We"

INTRODUCING
RICK & MARCY JACKSON

WE FIRST MET the Jacksons in 1997 after Parker Palmer suggested Jay and I drive north from our home in Portland, Oregon, where we worked at Lewis & Clark College at the time, to get acquainted with them. They had recently signed on to create the Center for Courage & Renewal, a nonprofit organization based on Parker's writings and work. Sitting in their "office," a separate building next to their country home on Bainbridge Island in Washington (which is a ferry ride away from Seattle), we were surrounded by towering walls of bookshelves with tempting collections of poetry, novels, art books, spiritual writings, and progressive theology. The Jacksons dished up warm, homemade apple pie as we discussed the formation of this new organization, dedicated to reconnecting souls and roles for educators, using the Circle of Trust process. We can't begin to capture the excitement Jay and I felt about this emerging possibility of a movement committed to offering the teachers we worked with something so healing and powerful, so needed.

On this day, we were invited into a friendship and the initiation of a community that turned out to infiltrate the root system of our spiritual formation and careers going forward. It also framed the lives of Marcy and Rick for the years ahead. Touched by their welcome, authenticity, and bright, intelligent presence, we couldn't help but wonder: How did we get so lucky?

A quarter of a century later, after sharing years of collaboration, leadership, travel, heartbreaks, and learning with them, we once again found ourselves on Bainbridge Island—now in their new environs, a planned living community near the little Northwest island town—to enter our interview process with these dear friends.

Rick and Marcy met at St. Olaf College in Northfield, Minnesota, in the Scandinavian Midwest, whose students call themselves Oles. They are always up for a good laugh at themselves and embody the paradox that wherever there is serious work going on, laughter is never far off.

They initially noticed each other during their first year in college when playing touch football. Afterward, they attended a folk dance and evening mixer, where Marcy approached Rick and told him that she needed a partner. He walked her back to the dorm, where they sat outside on a curb and chatted about Rick's travels in Europe. Marcy then hid from Rick for over a month because she was still in a long-term relationship with a boyfriend from high school, who was now attending a different college. This boyfriend was pressing her for a commitment, but she realized that the life ahead with him felt predictable. She was young and ready for excitement and adventure. A relationship with Rick promised a bigger life and a bigger dream, with his summer trekking in

Europe and plans for attending seminary. By Thanksgiving, she broke up with her boyfriend and dated Rick for the next three-and-a-half years. She sensed she could grow with Rick. When they graduated, with Rick heading to seminary and intentions to travel to Scotland, they thought they needed to get married to travel together. They realized that if they didn't commit to each other at this point, they would probably not stay together. You can guess what they decided to do, now forty-four years later.

The newlyweds moved a half-continent away from friends and family in their first year and confessed it was the worst year of their marriage. Their expectations and understanding of what comprised a loving relationship were inadequate, formed with overly romantic, gender-role-infused notions of what love is. As he was conditioned to do, Rick single-mindedly pursued his career goals and soon forgot their wedding anniversary. Marcy thought marriage was about creating a warm home for each other and making one another the priority. When the relationship failed to deliver on their expectations, they began to confront their problems. It was tough.

Rick's father didn't remember birthdays or anniversaries either. He talked to a male friend about handling these things, who wisely told him to write the dates down in his calendar. Marcy said, "In terms of 'me and we,' Rick was all about 'me.' His early career focused on making his mark, but we were missing each other, and having unspoken assumptions that got us into trouble. As we have gone through our lives, I have moved more towards the 'me' and Rick, more towards the 'we.' Rick had career success, and now his focus is back here. I feel empowered and free to go off and do some other things."

This theme of "me and we" is a tension and dynamic throughout the life of a relationship as we work on our individuation and pursue our callings and vocation. When people retire, they again negotiate the balance of "me and we" since they no longer go off to workplaces that, at one time, offered a regular pattern of leaving and returning each day. Rick and Marcy worked together, which created even more pressure on this issue for them.

Marcy said, "We didn't know the questions to ask. We didn't know how to fight. We saw somebody in marriage counseling who asked us what we wanted to get out of our marriage. He named an image that has endured, with Rick floating with his feet off the ground and my hand in his back pocket, my feet grounded. This speaks to Rick's propensity to think big and try on lots of ideas, while I am the practical one who helps him ground where he goes. We both have different but complementary ways of being and seeing the world, and our therapist helped us see this."

Rick continued, "We examined how both of us came from parents who had been married a long time, in Marcy's case, happily so. When I met them, I thought I had won the lottery. In my twenties, I came to the awareness of how unhappy my parents were. They continued to be disappointed together in a sixty-six-year marriage. The therapist suggested a session with my parents and that I tell my narcissistic mom that Marcy is the most important person to me. This was an essential part of my individuation, shifting from trying to please everyone to sorting out my priorities. I realized I wanted to make this marriage work, wanted to keep growing, noticed the way I think out loud, and needed to spend more time internally pondering. I needed to stop talking to allow that to happen."

As young as the Jacksons were, they had the wisdom to seek help and invest in their relationship. They drew on the Myers-Briggs Type Indicator and the Enneagram to explore their personality differences. They formed a couples' group, which stayed together for five years, where they openly discussed their concerns about sex, money, career balance, gender issues, etc. Looking back, they consider this group critical to what kept them together.

There is a saying that it takes a village to raise a child. You could also add that it takes a community to support a marriage, and many couples don't have one. Through the experience of conducting these interviews, Jay and I believe that couples in our culture receive scant attention and support.

Rick and Marcy's experiences confirmed what we noticed in the interviews and have experienced: relationships contain a dark gift. They take us to the painful places in ourselves that are in most need of transformation and healing. You are brought together for this work. It is as though a shadow can fall across the relationship based on cultural expectations, past family/childhood trauma, and the withholding and distancing behaviors we fall back on, which become entrenched patterns that erode the relationship if left unchecked.

"Rick might have done something that bothered me, and in the heat of some moment, I am trying to correct the situation and say to him, 'This is how you should do it. I see it this way.' Rick has said, in these moments, 'I don't hear your words, but your tone of voice. I am being scolded.' I am not aware of it but I am communicating judgment. Thus, I try to be more thoughtful of timing, tone of voice, or if I am trying to score points. That can be problematic. I have to work with my anger and my feelings and then calm them down enough for the messages to have a chance of getting through. I might not perceive that edge, but other people can feel it."

Numerous articles online regarding baby boomers point to the rise of divorce rates among older couples. If we don't engage in this difficult work of growing together, the failure to do so can break relationships apart.

Marcy concluded, "Love asks of us in long-term relationships to be truth-tellers to each other with as much kindness as possible; to become mirrors to what we can't see in ourselves, and mirror what is going on between us, thus facing things together. Playing different roles at different times, we ask, 'Why is that happening?' We talk through things and try to be encouraging as we face these things. It is about shadow work. To be vulnerable and honest with each other takes love and the belief your partner is mirroring this because they have your best interest in mind. There is an unwritten contract that we are together to become the most we can be and to become more whole, accepting all of who we are, both light and shadow.

"This role is true in close friendships too. Our love also makes me not want to be complacent and pretend that a difficult thing is not happening. What is currently occurring in our lives is intensely challenging, but in the midst of it, we have had more heart and soul-searching conversations and faced some things in ourselves. In any close relationship with someone I deeply love—Rick and others—I realize that part of why we are here is to help each other and be partners on the journey: to mirror, encourage, and challenge. Not everyone is up for or thinks they signed up for that. To me, it is some of the deeper meaning of what love is, to have each other's highest interest at heart."

Paradoxically, while our shadow qualities may be hard to love, the vulnerability we embrace to invite them in is lovable and bonding for a couple. It is in our vulnerability and openness, not our strengths and achievements, that we deeply connect with others.

As we continued with the interview, the theme of soul and role was soon with us again. As mentioned earlier, Rick and Marcy were co-founders and directors of the Center for Courage & Renewal. As they step back from this work, we asked them about what is bringing them alive now and where their sense of calling continues to draw them.

Rick began. "Having negotiated challenges with our adult kids, the death of my parents, and my sister's death, I have been absorbed in my family. To become an elder in my own family has been a bit of a surprising vocation. I am deeply loyal to my sister. I walked with her through years of living and dying of cancer."

Rick discussed the process of ending his official career and what was asked of him. "There has been quite a bit of leave-taking, including leaving my leadership role at the Center. I value 'honorable closure,' which can apply in any dimension of life. I am a slower leave-taker than I want to be. The YMCA leadership role faded slowly as well, regarding my identity. Right now, I am teaching, but I am ready to hand it off. I am asking, 'Okay, if there are things I'm doing that others can do, whose hands can I leave them in?' Offering my listening and advice in coaching conversations, I work with a handful of younger people who are in the fray. In many ways, I am in a 'neutral zone' before new beginnings, as defined by William Bridges. I have conversations about this with men friends where we talk about what is up with us, from the delight in being grandparents to not wanting it to be a full-time job. It is important to live my own life, not my children's. Travel I have always loved and have done quite a bit already. I hope to click that up more. I enjoy doing things with Marcy and learning together, including some retreat work."

Marcy added her story to what is calling her now. "When I retired, I joined boards. I was on a board for three months when I thought, 'I don't have it in me.' I resigned. I told them,

'You need people who are into this.' I feel much more impatient with things. How much of these meetings is busy work in the name of getting something done? Time is short, and I am asking if I am using my time well. I never liked the passion question, for it represents giving everything over to that one thing.

"My vocation now can be captured in three words: to create, to love, and to serve. The creativity piece is vital to me. I want to paint and engage in artistic expression, work with light and color, and create with other people. This is something I have to give. The love part is deeper and more layered now. Work demanded a lot of us; now, we are mainly sharing our love with our families and supporting our children. My definition of how to serve feels more spacious. It is the way I show up to other people."

Marcy is enrolled in a program called Warriors for the Human Spirit, designed by author Margaret Wheatley.[1] This training helps develop the qualities and skillful means necessary to protect and preserve the human spirit and the spirit of life. Marcy shared, "Warriors for the Human Spirit have only two 'weapons'—compassion and insight. We are in a time of collapse. The planet is showing all of those signs. How can I prepare myself and not add to the violence and fear? I need to deal with those things within myself. That is the training ground. Instead of focusing it out there, I have ample opportunity to deal with my deep feelings, intense anger, rage, and confusion within my own family system and with close friends. This training doesn't need to lead anywhere but is of value already. More close-in, I am restless and want to make a difference in a significant way. I am listening to that. Inner-generational work has had a lot of meaning. That is part of my future."

Discerning the next steps in life is an ongoing process. The Quakers have an adage that the door that closes shows the way as much as the door that opens. Aging is a time for listening closely for natural endings—like Marcy's experiences with board work or Rick handing over teaching—and for what is now bringing us alive. It is deeply personal, individual work. No one can determine your call for you at any stage of life.

We found the Jacksons especially wise regarding discernment practices. Marcy began, "Great question about how we make decisions! Rick and I come at things differently. I first have to go through my own discernment process. Then it is about us coming together and creating the space and time to listen to each other, to hear where the obstacles and opportunities are in the situation. We are often on the same page, and it doesn't take a lot of conversations, as it is an easy recognition. Even in our spiritual lives, there was a time when I first started meditation at Spirit Rock, the Jack Kornfield meditation center in California; I would get up very early, sit and meditate each day. Back home, one morning, Rick suddenly pads in and put his cushion next to me, and I knew that this wasn't going to work. This is my space. I felt that it was wonderful he wanted to do this, but I knew I needed meditation time to start the day alone, that it was critical to me. Then we could talk and share. I now meditate in my room, he sits out in the living room, and then we have our tea and talk. This is a daily thing to intentionally sense what is needed while honoring our differences."

Rick continued, "I agree. The 'me and we' has been a changing dance. As a couple, we are both alone, then together, rather than the mush of endless togetherness. We each have energy fields and ways of calming the waters. We've had to learn to lead and then follow with each other. I see discernment as thoughtful decision-making, a spiritual discipline, and a practice. In recent years working with the L'Arche community, an organization that serves the mentally challenged through establishing group housing, I noticed they take discernment very seriously. There is a lot of mutuality and it is very respectful. It is such an important way of leading and is seldom practiced well. Discernment is the right word to be inviting us to explore. We need to be respectful of the deep individuality and interiority of each other. We must have respect for each other's leadings. When we are not respectful, the results are less."

Marcy noted, "There is a process of listening for spiritual guidance that comes in as a voice or knowing where I feel certainty. All of a sudden, I know what I need to know. I've grown to trust it. It isn't always right, but it gives me something if I have done the listening. With this kind of knowing, we have made some powerful decisions, like moving to the West Coast; we felt called somehow, even though we had family, friends, and good jobs in Minnesota. The actual reason we moved didn't appear to us clearly for several years. We would not have started the Center for Courage & Renewal had we not moved. We wouldn't have done something so out of the box had we not moved, to lead a start-up non-profit. The guidance told us to move, but not why we should. That came later."

Time and age call us to care deeply for our adult children, who grow up and develop their own lives, with all of the joys and challenges life presents. Both of the Jacksons' daughters live nearby in Seattle, so we asked Marcy and Rick if they have any wisdom to share about relationships with adult children.

Marcy began. "A big learning for me, inner learning, is the importance of knowing what is mine and what is theirs. I can companion them, and support them, but I can't do their work. It requires me to see them as whole people. I also have to look at my behavior as a mom and where it might have contributed to some of their issues. I don't spend a lot of time beating myself up about that. We did the best we could with what we knew at the time. Our parents did the same thing. I truly want to be clear about where my role and relationship extend and where I am over-functioning and enabling. I want to see my daughters as whole and capable of finding their own answers in their own time."

Rick added, "I can slide towards over-functioning in my relationships with my daughters. This is part of my work. Love includes a commitment to look for wholeness and trust in it. We do things we aren't proud of and are all so human. Welcome to the human race."

Marcy said, "Sometimes it's just continuing to show up. It is not about what we are doing or saying, but how we are. There is so much overlay of baggage and unintended messaging going on in such close relationships with adult children. I need to look at our dynamics as clearly as I can. I ask myself, 'Where do I need to be responsible for my feelings, let myself be okay with feeling angry, disappointed, and sadness, but not lay these feelings on others?' It has felt like an inner journey and a huge teacher. And continuing to model that we have a sense of joy, meaning, and adventure in our own lives, and the things we want to pursue."

Rick and Marcy jointly concluded with how much they cherish being able to hop a ferry and spend a day with their grandchildren in Seattle.

Our final question invites reflection about what couples hope their legacy will be. In a way, this question seemed premature, for the Jacksons are still fully engaged in the world, working in Europe and South Africa leading Circle of Trust retreats. Still, they did have much to say about legacy.

Marcy noted that their children and family are their most significant legacy, created through their partnership, which will be passed on to the next generation. As co-founders of the Center for Courage & Renewal, they see that their legacy includes giving form to how Circles of Trust have been shared in the world and will continue, no matter what happens to the Center in the future. When they began leading retreats and directing the Center, they modeled how as a couple, they could partner in meaningful ways with their different gifts—never perfect, but making a real contribution in a world that is struggling with broken relationships. They hope their legacy includes people acknowledging that they were a good team who respected each other, and worked to serve others, without being overly enmeshed.

We wish to end this chapter with their responses to the question, "What do you hope your children will say about you?"

Rick began with, "I hope my daughters can say, 'Dad was there for me—both cheering on the sidelines at a soccer match, graduations, and performances, and also when it was difficult. He extended unconditional love.' I also hope they know I was grateful for life, whatever its measure in years. Finally, I hope they would say that I provided a source of affirmation in confidence that no matter how difficult and dark life can be, it is a gift to be celebrated."

Marcy concluded, "Being a mother was such a primary and important role for me. While nurturing, holding, and comforting were hugely important, they didn't come first. There is a gender piece in this for me. I want them to see that I showed up as fully as I could, tried to live and act with integrity, and was not afraid to have hard conversations. I hope they know that I cherished family and friends, work, and meaningful relationships; that was what life was all about for me. As a woman with daughters, I want them to have a model of a woman living into her own fullness, including being a mom, which is what I wanted from my mother. I know I have strong daughters. I want them to thrive and love the fullness of their lives."

*... the world cannot be discovered by a journey of miles,
no matter how long, but only by a spiritual journey,
a journey of one inch, very arduous and humbling
and joyful, by which we arrive at the ground
at our feet and learn to be at home.*

WENDELL BERRY

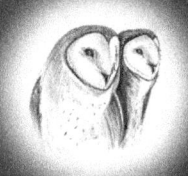

Blessed is the couple who
practices the Sabbath through
the daily bread of devotion,
mindfulness, and prayer,
for they shall find Home.

BLESSED IS THE COUPLE WHO
Practices the Sabbath

INTRODUCING
KAREN NOORDHOFF & DAVID HAGSTROM

ON A BLUE-BIRD-SKY summer morning in Sisters, Oregon, we pulled into "The Clearing," Karen and David's cabin in the woods. We had to brake for a flock of wild turkeys trotting across the driveway with outstretched, skinny necks leading them towards the backyard; they nervously strutted en masse, making a squawking racket, and settled down to scratch for seeds and bugs on the lawn. Up the hill, a mother mule deer and her fawn glanced up to stare at us as they nibbled grass. A separate hand-built writing studio offered a refuge for scores of golden-mantled squirrels that darted in and out from their holey homes under the cabin, steadily undermining its foundation. To the left of the driveway, down the hill, we gazed at the labyrinth, lined with blooming lavender plants, lava rocks, and a restful view of the distant Cascade mountains. Attached to the side of the garage was a greenhouse, its roof collapsed in by last winter's "snowmageddon." Karen and David call their cabin "The Clearing" because they like to get clear out of the city of Portland, where they also own a home, to enjoy the quieter rhythms of nature and the pure air. The Clearing provides a sanctuary for their souls.

We have a history with Karen and David. When they moved to Portland from Alaska, David found his way to Lewis & Clark College, where Jay was then the academic dean of the graduate school, and I was on the faculty. Jay instantly hired David, whose reputation as a school leader and college educator preceded him. Karen worked across town at Portland State University in teacher education. The four of us became facilitators for the Center for Courage & Renewal, and while still working at Lewis & Clark College, David and I taught classes together and co-led scores of Circle of Trust retreats for many years. We have been blessed with their friendship and have lived in each other's neighborhoods for over thirty years in Portland and Central Oregon. The interview process offered us yet another opportunity to enjoy these two old souls.

Karen and David met while working for the National College of Education in Evanston, Illinois, now over thirty-seven years ago. David occupied the role of undergraduate dean, and Karen served as a representative of the Faculty Welfare Committee. David, a runner at the time, searched for flowers along his route each morning. He would proudly present a bouquet of "found flowers" to Karen when they would congregate at Lighthouse Park on Lake Michigan before work. They fell in love and eventually moved to Alaska to continue to build a life together.

How they decided to marry is more dramatic. While still courting, David was diagnosed with a cancerous brain tumor and informed that the physicians would perform surgery to remove it, but with no guarantee that he would survive. They told him he should make final preparations. A chaplain and friend asked him, "If you live through this, what do you have to live for?"

David immediately replied that he would marry Karen. The chaplain said that he should remember his intention during the fourteen-hour surgery and, "Whatever you do, don't go into the light." David survived to marry Karen, and she has remained "side by side" with him through many ongoing health challenges over time.

After the brain surgery, David was in the hospital for three weeks and lost most of his hearing and his ability to talk and walk. He said, "Even with those difficulties, Karen stayed right with me. She was spectacular. As a result of many years of physical therapy, my current condition is best described as follows: I have a completely dead right ear, limited hearing in the left, a right eyelid that will not close, vocal cord dysfunction, and other mobility limitations. However, my current medical team often announces my arrival at our meetings in this way: 'Oh good, here comes The Walking Wonder.' Their greeting always cheers me up!"

What we realized about David and Karen is something so simple and basic that it is easy to overlook its profound nature: these two are helpmates. Hopefully, all couples are mates that assist one another as needed, but Karen and David stand out to us as beautiful examples. Helping sometimes comes in the form of caregiving, as described above. Each morning, upon awakening, David greets Karen with, "Good morning! How can I assist you today?" This invites the spirit of mutuality, a crucial quality for couples to thrive.

When we asked Karen and David how they demonstrate their love for each other, David disclosed how "the story lady appears," recalling when his fourth-grade teacher took his class to the library so they could check out books. She would then read them a story at 2 p.m. each week. Since then, he has loved being read to, so at bedtime, Karen reads a story or book to him for about twenty minutes before falling asleep. David thinks this is pretty much the best part of the day. He also noted that Karen takes walks with him as far as he can endure, even though she can walk much faster and farther.

Karen recalled David's expressing his love to her during a tough winter season when she had overcommitted to facilitating Circle of Trust retreats in a compressed time period; she felt a sense of chronic pressure. She owned that she was constantly on edge. The irony of the situation troubled her; she was leading retreats on deep listening and leading from the soul, while she felt unhinged at home and out of integrity with her own inner needs. Over these six weeks, David observed her situation but didn't try to fix it or make it (or her) different. He held a compassionate space for what she was going through, using his focus and energy to keep them both together. She cited this as an example of how David was a loving helpmate when she most needed it, an expression of mutuality. He put aside his desire to be closer to Karen and let her undergo her ordeal. Sometimes giving our partners space to get our work done is the most helpful, loving thing we can do.

Some call love in the later years "antique love." Antique love is often expressed without words. A penetrating look from a loved one can even save a life! Karen's attunement and careful gaze saved David's life when he had a severe internal bleeding episode that turned into a life-threatening event.

Reading aloud together in bed one night, David discovered a pool of blood beneath him. Although he briefly resisted, Karen called 911. An ambulance arrived, and they soon found themselves in the emergency room of Portland's Good Samaritan Hospital. Upon arrival, David and Karen endured the admissions process and initial assessment phase. They then sat helplessly as David lay on a gurney in the intake room, awaiting more medical attention. Time was passing, and it seemed nothing was happening. Meanwhile, Karen noticed David's condition worsening as he was losing all color; he was slipping away, and she knew he was in grave danger. Through sheer will and a bold confrontation with the staff, she found an emergency room nurse who quickly confirmed her worst suspicions. David was rushed off to surgery, followed by what turned out to be a lengthy stay at the hospital. Because Karen was attuned to David, she knew in her body, mind, and soul that she needed to act quickly. She also grasped she wasn't ready or willing to lose him. Karen's attention saved David's life.

When in their presence, this couple's love of beauty, travel, and learning is tangible. It is as though they carry many geographies and adventures within them. We met them just as they moved to Oregon from Alaska, trailing visions of Northern Lights, deep cold, snow, avalanches, and Alaskan Native sensibilities behind them. Moving to urban Portland was a tough transition, especially for David. Many couples must negotiate different needs regarding where to live and work, sometimes practicing mutuality in fundamentally challenging ways.

When we asked them what most tested their love, the following story emerged. David spoke about his profound kinship with Alaska, her people, and all of the stimulating escapades it offered them. "In Alaska, every day was an adventure. Rural schools' leadership took me into all of the villages. Karen's work with the Teach Alaska program was full of adventure, too, which moved us forward every day with exciting, surprising, new challenges." They traveled in small planes to the villages and people. David even survived being buried by an avalanche when cross-country skiing alone. This was indeed a season of adventure for them.

One of the final Alaskan escapades occurred when David lost a campaign to become the commissioner of education for Alaska. His disappointment was quite a traumatic descent for David and required them both to look at what to do next. Karen received an invitation to work at Portland State University. Previously, out of a desire to support Karen, David had told her, "I will be a trailing spouse when something opens up for you."

David explained, "I thought, well, I can do that, move to Portland. Yet I was so distraught. Karen and others asked if I might want to send out resumes in Oregon. I was stubborn, elected not to make calls, and simply drove alone from Alaska to our new home. I say that because I was not very good about this change." David came to Portland without a job and wandered around the noisy urban downtown near their rented apartment, conversing with parking lot attendants. He felt in exile, angry, and lost. Eventually, he found his way to Lewis & Clark College, where Jay hired him to teach in the educational leadership program. This transition was not an easy time for them as a couple. All couples go through tough patches, as Karen says. This was one of them.

Karen noted, "'Test' is a good word. I realize that couples must learn to accept that we have different stories about the same event. I want to say, 'No, the actual story is . . .' Now I know that people have different stories about the same incident that we must live with. Just let the different stories be. My story about our move to Portland is that when finishing my doctoral work, David told me to get a job that will fit who I am, and we would go there. Being self-absorbed at that stage, I took it literally. When he lost the commissioner position, I got this job in Portland, and I thought we would take it and act on this promise. David didn't want to leave Alaska. Over time I have seen how difficult that was for him. He was wandering around inside of himself and not knowing where to go. That year was a test. It was hard for him and hard for me to start a new job. We weren't very nice to each other. This was a test of our love, and we got through it. The other tests have been dealing with David's health challenges, but we found that those tests cemented us, in a bonding sense."

In realizing that they had different stories about this life transition that took them from the wilds of Alaska to the urban center of Portland, she doesn't say, "I am right, and you are wrong." She just wisely makes room for their different truths. Being right, and proving you're right, doesn't do anything for a couple. It is a wisdom move, a loving move, to make room for "two truths" about the same situation.

David concluded these reflections about their years in Alaska with, "Our sense of adventure is different now. The current adventure is about growing older together." A friend of his, Dave Holloway, told him when he turned seventy, "You are now entering the time of gifts. This is the time when you will be able to sing your true songs. You know the job stuff is gone, money worries, gone. You can be who your soul has wanted you to be all along." Now that is a true adventure!

David pulled out a book and read his favorite quote from Jean Vanier, founder of the L'Arche community. It speaks to this new freedom and adventure of aging and the kind of presence he now offers himself and others. "There are old people with a child's heart who have used their freedom from function and rest to find a new youth. They have the wonder of a child but the wisdom of maturity as well. They have integrated their years of activity and so can live without being attached to power. Their freedom of heart and their acceptance of limitations and weakness makes them people whose radiance illuminates the whole community."[1]

Karen was born twelve years later than David. We were curious about what their age difference is like for them and how they can teach others about working creatively with age differences. When younger, age differences are generally not that noticeable, but as the years progress, a couple can encounter more of a contrast.

"I think people were worried about our age difference when we married, especially my family," Karen revealed. "We were well aware of it but oblivious in other ways. We were in love and had a strong sense we were meant to be together. In a way, I have always been waiting for this stage of life we are in now. This is the phase when we would recognize what this age difference would mean to us. What it has allowed me, in thirty-plus years, is the opportunity to witness and learn from David how one person moves through different phases of life. While not exactly a generation apart, twelve years is enough to situate us in different stages at various times of our marriage. I get to watch David make the bends around the big zero birthdays, and witness how he has worked to become his own advocate for health. When he is not here, I will have his voice informing me about the ways he would work through the health challenges, or remind me of daily routines that are healthful, and about taking time for contemplation."

David reflected a positive perspective as well. "I have felt quite fortunate about the age difference. Yes, there is a twelve-year difference, but we like many of the same songs, books, and practices, as though there isn't that big of a difference at all between us. I wonder if some of the difficulties with my health are a burden for Karen. I am sure they are. But I am not very aware of how much of a burden my health issues are for her. That has to do with her way of giving and caring. So yes, there is an age difference, but it hasn't been debilitating, from my point of view."

In the spirit of approaching aging as a new adventure, when you listen to their stories and their choices regarding how to spend their time, Karen and David focus on the new freedom from the roles they previously occupied by attending to their creative lives.

David said, "I go back to when I was eight years old. It was such a beautiful, pure, innocent time for me. Believe it or not, I feel, at age eighty-three, close to age eight when I played in the dirt. Between eight and eight-three, there were just a number of things that took me away from the way I was at eight and how I felt free. Things like wounds, physical wounds; I completely accept those wounds. There are no trappings now, no need for power, no intention to have my name in the lights, nor prove anything, like climb the career ladder. Doing all of that, I realized my false self entered the picture. The best example of my false self was when I ran a campaign to be commissioner of education in Alaska. That wasn't my true self, and I've realized that, even though it was tough losing. I am now to the point I have integrated all that has happened in my life and combined some things with wisdom."

Part of the grace of aging is this immense freedom to explore our creative natures. While Karen was a writer in an academic setting throughout her career, her writing now focuses on her own story, often discouraged in scholarly publications. She is now free to go creatively where she wants to go.

David can no longer work as much in their yard from morning until night, caring for their property in Sisters, Oregon. He disclosed how he spends his time instead. "I look forward to a summer of writing and digging deeper into all manner of things we value. I want to spend a lot of time in the writing house. My passion currently, and for the past two years, is captured in the book I am writing, *Messengers of Encouragement.*[2] I am trying to find just the right questions people can ask one another that would encourage us. This is a very exciting journey for me."

David picked up a picture of a stone farmhouse in Provence, France. It's a place David's physician gifted them to use while recovering from his heart surgery. They now travel there for three months at a time, whenever they can. He explained, "The fabric market in France was inspiring to Karen. I found helpful scenarios in France as well and have written one essay about how everyday people encourage each other in cafes in Paris. On Armistice Day, which marks the end of World War I, I witnessed the president of France, Emmanuel Macron, after giving a formal presentation to thank the veterans in France for saving the country, walk across the street and shake hands with all of the people watching the event, asking them questions about the meaning of the day for them. He shook 200 hands, asked questions, and listened. I thought, 'This is amazing.' I thought it was over, but he walked another block and did it again. I am finding one story after another about encouragement." In this story, their love of France, and passion for their creative lives, coalesce as a way of life.

Like many of the *Side by Side* couples, Karen and David embrace the value of establishing a "Sabbath" in their relationship for rest, sharing, prayer and meditation, discernment practices, working through conflicts, and spiritual readings to enrich their inner growth, alone and together.

"We started a practice last year of gathering around 6 p.m.; we call our 'wine time.' We start with a prayer," said David. "We want to both pray and learn about compassion, so we are reading a book by Joyce Rupp on this theme.[3] Afterwards, we have glasses of wine available."

Karen continued. "We have a number of different places and experiences for our literal Sabbath time zone at 6 p.m. This space here in Sisters, Oregon, offers a sanctuary away from city life. We feel a sense of being rooted, grounded, and clear. There is a literal and internal open land to clear away what is crowding us. We also have a sanctuary from the sanctuary, the writing house, and separate studio space to retreat to on this land. That is a place we can go more deeply into creativity and understanding." They also consider their travels to France, Alaska, and camping on the nearby Metolius River in Oregon as other "sanctuary sites."

You are probably sensing that Karen and David savor quiet, beautiful places in nature. They are introverted, deep, grounded people who know how to protect their inner landscapes. They've grown into the wisdom of allowing things time and exercising this ability with their conflicts and discernment processes.

"I like the saying, 'pulling the shades down around us,'" David noted. "Creating a sanctuary for our conflicts means pulling the shades down until we feel restored enough to go out and be active in the world. We don't pull down the shades between us but around us. We are plodders. We are earth folks. We inch along until we get things figured out. That is a mark of our relationship."

Karen added, "There is this song, 'Shingle by Shingle,' by Eric Bibb, we first heard in the period before my mother died. This song represents our relationship. We patch up our roof a shingle at a time."

Karen described how they used "pulling down their shades" to tenderly plod through the season of her mother's death. "An example of a rough patch was the period before my mother died in 2015. It wasn't so much a rough patch between us, but for us. That summer, there were not only physical clues of mom's decline, but I had strong feelings of foreboding.

We canceled a sabbatical trip to France for the fall; it was all a big brew and a mess of emotions. In my prayers, I asked, 'God. I could use your help right now. I could use help being kind right now.' Leading up to Mom's death, I didn't know who would pray for me when she died. She was a prayer. Mom was a person of personal faith with a deep prayer life. After her death, a switch turned, and my personal prayer life activated. David and I started saying an out-loud prayer at wine time. Now, that prayer always initiates this time together. When in a rough patch, we are bolder and inclined to pray directly for the two of us. This is an adventure. We are sorting it out now."

Many couples reported how much they have in common in terms of interests and values but are quite different from one another in terms of their personalities. Karen explained, "My natural inclination is to notice what is not quite right. What is missing in a situation is the best way to put it. It is just the way my mind works since my sense of analysis is inclined toward evaluation and critique. For example, when we arrive at the Clearing, on our first evening, sitting out on the front porch, David is usually waxing romantic about how great it is and the remarkable beauty; I see the weeds and what needs to be done and repaired. This is a tension between us that is unsolvable. We just continue to live with it."

David noted, "I used to react. 'So Karen, you want me to cut those weeds right now, with a glass of wine in hand?' I have modified my response to something like, 'I will take care of the weeds tomorrow.' It is an issue but not a terrible problem. That is how I have learned to live with it."

Karen responded, "I don't mean it that way, for it is not about me giving a direction. Now I can say, 'This is David,' who tends to personalize things. For him, he hears it as a direction. I now know this about David, for it has to do with being relationship-oriented. He hears a lot of stuff personally."

When we began this project, we were most curious about the intersection of aging and spirituality. Karen and David's partnership has interwoven these two themes with their age differences, health challenges, their deep faith journeys alone and together, and Sabbath times for rest, prayer, and soulful communication. We end with two final stories that, once again, find their origins in their adventures in Alaska. We share them as examples of two people, living side by side, devoted to one another in Spirit.

Karen told the story of joining a church community. "At the Saint Matthew's Episcopal Church in Fairbanks, Alaska, the priest was new to his role. He didn't know the appropriate service for people who were non-Episcopalian but practicing Christians wanting to join the church. We loved that he wore red tennis shoes under his robe and had such a connection to everyone. Eventually, we settled on an Affirmation of Baptism, performed by the bishop of Alaska, a Choctaw Indian. The bishop wore this stunningly beautiful beaded robe and carried a staff with an eagle feather. It felt mystical when he spoke to the two of us in front of the congregation. Without meeting us before, he named who we are, not just surface things, but David's capacity for encouragement and leadership, and regarding me, support to let the quiet joy come out from within. He spoke from a place of mystery and inspiration from God, and we had an incredible experience of the Holy Spirit moving in us for forty-eight hours after the ceremony. The joy we experienced was unlike any joy before."

David followed up with a story of a brush-with-death experience.

"I visited almost every rural village in Alaska on floatplanes, little four-seaters—a pilot, me, and two other people. One time we were flying to Dillingham—or, in the native language, Curyung, a city in southwestern Alaska. The director of the Alaska Department of Education was next to me, along with a public health nurse. I was representing the University of Alaska. When we got close to Dillingham, the pilot said, 'I've lost my autopilot process, and we are in a white-out. The only thing I can do is find the river with a visual sighting, and then we will be able to make it in. We'll just have to land and take our chances if I can't.' We had a half tank of gas left, then an eighth, and we were still not finding the river. When down to a trace of gas, the three passengers and pilot just decided to sing 'Onward Christian Soldiers.' I held the pilot's hand. When we finished the last note, the river appeared. We were totally prepared that this might be the end, but it wasn't. The director said, 'What a mystical experience that was. Won't we be friends forever!'"

This story stands as a metaphor and a reminder for all of us aging: we never know when the moment might come when the autopilot system that has guided us will fail, and we begin to run out of gas. It is in those times that we turn to each other, hold hands, and sing. It will be our time to follow the river home.

This seems to be the harsh secret of time: the more our bodies and minds are carved out, the more brightly we shine.

MARK NEPO

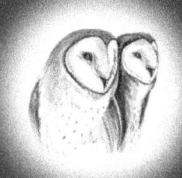

Blessed is the couple who
extends mercy and forgiveness,
for they shall be relieved of
resentment and harsh judgment.

BLESSED IS THE COUPLE WHO
Extends Mercy & Forgiveness

INTRODUCING
MICHAEL & EILEEN HEATON

WE DIDN'T NEED to travel far for our interview with Michael and Eileen Heaton, for at the time, we lived in the same town: Bend, Oregon. While we didn't know them well, we had recently taken a class they offered on the ancient wisdom of the Enneagram. This tool has been very helpful to our marriage, especially in terms of understanding our differences and shadows. Eileen served as the choir director at our church; her musical gifts and beautiful voice are stunning. Michael was the board chair for the Sacred Art of Living Center where I had worked, yet we had never sat down for a conversation. Jay and I were enthralled when we learned about their creative lives and history, beginning with the story of when they fell in love.

When they met, Michael worked as a professional stage director in New York City. Eileen auditioned for and got a part during an open audition for *My Fair Lady* in an equity theater, with 200 to 300 people trying out. They were ages twenty-seven and twenty-nine, and both recovering from ending long-term relationships. Eileen, married to a dancer, divorced when she learned he was gay. She reflects on how she felt when she met Michael. "Theater brought us together. I felt as though he admired me. He told me I was the most beautiful, talented girl, and to this day, there is a sense of admiration between us. I feel the same way now as when he hired me. He is so talented. He knows what he is doing, can take charge, be creative, artistic, etc." When two people share a similar calling and vocation, there is often a powerful bond and soul recognition.

From the beginning, hard work and a capacity to manifest dreams through numerous creative endeavors defined their relationship. They started rehearsing for *My Fair Lady* in August 1978, began dating in February, and then married in August 1979. Michael said, "We fell in love, got married, and almost immediately became business partners. In Jersey City, for $20,000, we bought and renovated a row house. We worked eight to twelve hours a day. There was one bathtub, so we watched TV while the other person took a bath."

Michael and Eileen worked together for a while in a repertory in Myrtle Beach. "We always worked together. It is a thread. We are excellent partners when we have a project together. Things go smoothly."

However, it's no secret that life in show business is taxing on relationships. Their theater days hit hard times when the AIDS epidemic devastated the country. The small theaters on the edges went non-union due to the sharp increase in healthcare costs, and many jobs dried up. Eileen and Michael were also growing tired of airports, being away from home, and the insidious ways their work took them apart. As a director, Michael's job was over just as Eileen's, as an actress, began. They realized this was not what they wanted for their marriage.

Eileen cited a quiet moment of reckoning upon returning from a long summer away to their little house across the river from Manhattan. When they walked in the door, they discovered all of the house plants were dead, and the candles on their mantle had melted from the heat. Their relationship felt this way too. They realized it was time to pivot, and wondered what else they might do with their creative lives and careers. They knew that they wanted to work together. Michael thought, "People like my cooking. Eileen can run the front of the house. Let's open a restaurant!" So that is just what they did. They opened and operated a sixty-seat restaurant and bed-and-breakfast over the next ten years.

At this point, Eileen and Michael weren't sure their relationship would last, for the years in the theater had taken a toll. By now, they had moved out of the first stage of a relationship, which can feel like sharing a paradise on a tropical island, where couples often experience a deep soul connection and sexual passion for one another but don't really know each other. Now, they were in the second stage, more like a desert, with the dry, trying territory where you question your commitment. Now that you know each other, a period of doubting can set in. *Do I want to spend a lifetime with this person? Do I like this person?* This stage can last a long time and can be considerably painful and even lonely, filled with a sense of loss and even failure.

In Eileen's words, "Both of us were so sure we weren't going to stay together. We wondered, who would leave whom first? I had a sense of really wanting to feel I had a life partner. I wanted to know that what we had was solid, and I could invest in this, and there would be no out. The hard work of renovating buildings was an outward sign of what we were trying to do on the inside. Can we do this together? Be exhausted together? Set up a feeling of togetherness as though we had created an anchor we could move out from and not pull up?"

Eileen trusted Michael to be capable, and she knew he would work hard to create their next dream. Michael shared, "I always thought she trusted me, which was big for me. I knew we could open a restaurant. I had waited tables, but that is all I knew. So I found a seminar for training on how to do it and learning things like pricing a menu. Eileen just trusted me. That is part of our love and bond. I never felt starting this restaurant was a burden or an obligation, or only on me."

They were in it together and lived into their commitment to each other in the process. Eileen and Michael moved to the Midwest, where they reinvented their lives. In their thirties, these years were high points of hosting festivals, enjoying lots of friends, and being on a creative roll.

When we asked them to discuss how they show love to one another, Michael didn't hesitate to offer this story. "In Myrtle Beach, Eileen collected press releases and made a scrapbook for us of my shows, but she also mailed pieces back to my parents. She assumed, 'Of course, they would want to know this.' They didn't know what to do, but it meant a lot to me."

Eileen described something that occurred much later in their relationship. "The biggest thing Michael did for me is he stopped drinking. He became available in ways he wasn't before. This was monumental, his being more available, accompanied by more development for him. As a result, Michael became more comfortable and relaxed with himself. That was a pivotal time for us, the greatest gift he ever gave me!"

Michael credits Eileen for saving his life. "Without Eileen, I would not be anywhere, on any path. Had we not met, I would have stayed in New York, continued to be a director, made a living, drank and smoked too much, and been lucky to be alive at sixty-nine. This doesn't even cover the whole spiritual journey she opened up for me. One of the biggest surprises is that I am alive. Part of the blessing with Eileen is that she put up with and loved me through drinking too much for many years. I have been sober for eighteen years, half of our relationship. I was a functioning alcoholic for the first half of our time together."

Their story highlights the importance of partners supporting each other in the difficult work of addressing addictions, trauma, and wounds. Addictions arrest development and, if not treated, wreak havoc on relationships. It's likely that most of us have one form or another of reliance on unhealthy habits unconsciously developed to avoid our pain. Many of us recreate and act out our unfinished business from childhood in our relationships with our partners. At the very core, this unfinished business is how the spiritual work presents itself to us and where we can heal, alone and together.

Michael and Eileen had very different family backgrounds. Eileen grew up in a large, loving, Catholic family. In her words, "There were nine of us, with seven babies coming in nine years. I was the youngest of four girls, and it was hard for me because I was sure my mom wanted a boy. I felt I had to prove myself in the household by being helpful and taking on the mother's role. I imitated Mom and judged her critically. She worked her butt off for us. They were both musicians. Mom began as a professional singer and sang in Dad's band. My Dad was big and very theatrical. Every one of us became musicians, playing instruments. There was a cacophony of energy in our house. Life was so fun and lively, but it could be scary; it felt out of control. We never missed meals together when the chaos would stop, and we would be at the table. Many big events, church, holidays, and holy days were all celebrated as a family. I did learn a real sense of how to get along with people. We lived in a 1939 Tudor house with one bathroom. Nine kids negotiated the bathroom and shared beds. I benefited from this incredible legacy and learned how to be kind and to be a caretaker. My mother showed tenderness, but we all had abandonment issues. She simply had too many to take good care of us. Now I understand how attentive she was."

In contrast, Michael noted, "My father was in the Navy during World War II. Considered highly successful in his family, he was the oldest of five, but his life was screwed up. After football season, he was off to war to save the world. When he came home, there was no job, no aspirations, and no one telling him what to do. He met my mom at twenty-three, and they had me. Some fellow said to him, 'Oh Jim, join the reserves,' which he did, and then Korea happened, and he was called back up and was away for another two years. My sister came along. Then, he returned as an alcoholic. Mom worked nights at a hospital. With Dad, an alcoholic, and a passive-aggressive mother, they scared the crap out of me. I was disappointed in my father. His idea of being a father was to make money, pay the mortgage, and function, but show no signs of love or even kindness. Those things I was left to discover for myself."

As noted throughout these interviews, many men are working to overcome their "father wounds." Attempting to redefine masculinity in ways that are more holistic and life-giving, Michael leads men's groups designed to free them from these anti-intimacy, toxic male roles. As an elder now, he wants to leave a different legacy for himself and for the men who follow.

Eileen always assumed she would have children. When they were shocked to discover that she was infertile, this became another time for pivoting in their relationship. They went into a period of medical testing and decided not to push nature. She was healthy, and she didn't want to undergo invasive and dangerous procedures. This decision was a turning point in their marriage. They realized there would be no family; now, their world was the two of them. "This is just us having a life together," Eileen said.

But infertility was a profound loss for Eileen. "I had a sense of failure. How could I not get pregnant? I cried about it, but when talking to my mom, she said, 'Oh, Eileen. I don't need you to have a baby.' I could be who I am and have the life I am having. This turned our marriage inward."

In time, Michael and Eileen moved to Bend, Oregon, opened another popular restaurant, and eventually pivoted towards other endeavors, including nonprofit work for Michael and for Eileen, teaching, directing, and performing music, and creating a spiritual direction practice. Together, they discovered and studied the Enneagram. A complex, nuanced system, the Enneagram works with the structure of the personality that sheds the light of understanding onto oneself and others. Using this tool, they began to consult with organizations and teach classes based on the system. It also became an essential lens for them as a couple and for the ongoing work going deeper in understanding each other.

"We spent half of our marriage teaching the Enneagram system to others," said Michael. "It is a huge tool for understanding Eileen's Point One, an anger and body type. Realizing she isn't angry at me is very helpful, as is understanding the complexities of our personalities and differences. Not putting responsibility for her anger on myself is very helpful, realizing that this is Eileen's anger and issue, not mine. If I can be the best me, I can mirror her anger back to her. I am a fear type (Point Six) and in the headspace. She is sensitive to my aggression coming from my fear. Some fears are real, but most are made up. We can ask, 'What is it about?'"

It's helpful for couples to discover tools, a common language, and skills to negotiate their conflicts. The Enneagram is exceedingly useful in these areas.

Eileen noted, "When he became less reactive to my anger, that became the mirror. The mirror appeared because he wasn't actively trying to do anything about my anger. I try to name his fear for him as well. I can ask him, 'Am I making you afraid?' There will be times I am mirroring it, and this is effective. When we are not enmeshed, we are more helpful to each other. Then we are not getting caught in each other's shadows."

Eileen and Michael's capacity for standing back from each other's reactivity so they can mirror for each other what they see is invaluable, one of the greatest gifts we can give to our partners. Who else does this for you? Without a trustworthy mirror, it is very difficult to grow.

As a One on the Enneagram, Eileen disclosed, "I have a strong knowing of what we should eat, buy, and do. I try to soften myself around these opinions. I am usually right, but I know I am irritating to others. I wake up in the morning with my list of what I want to do or how I want to buy something. I often want fancy things, but Michael won't buy them. This strong inner sense of knowing, well, it won't change." Type One on the Enneagram tends to be perfectionistic, adheres to strict rules, has integrity, and is clear about what is important to them.

As a Six on the Enneagram, Michael said, "My experience with the Enneagram as a mental type has not, nor will it, change the fact that I have conversations in my head, and I don't always include Eileen in them early enough. A decision makes sense to me, but it is not clear to her. This is an ongoing issue."

We were curious about how Michael and Eileen, as people of faith, included Spirit in their times of conflict. Eileen said, "This morning, both of these patterns showed up. This is fresh. As we encounter a conflict, I try to say to myself, 'What is happening here?' That question is like a call to Spirit. Why are we back in this place, beating this dead horse again? I could not communicate what was going on inside of me, and he couldn't hear me. So I asked: 'What did I just trigger in him?' The call to Spirit is the call on my inner observer. I couldn't get there this morning. I am left with the question, and it helps me not feel personally hurt by what is just said. It is still perplexing, and I ask, 'Why again?' The question is the bridge to a new perspective. This morning it didn't work. We had to shift."

Michael added, "This morning, I did feel that Spirit asked, 'What is going on?' Spirit reminded me that there are choices. I said politely, 'This isn't going anyplace.' I followed that. It didn't work too well. Spirit helped me review and own what was mine in it."

In the autumn of our lives, tending our health is added to this inner workload. In a spirit of partnership, Eileen and Michael address their physical challenges with the same honesty and capacity as they employed when producing plays and opening restaurants.

Eileen began, "One of the biggest surprises at this time of life is how much our attention has turned to the caretaking of our bodies. You don't know until you know. I realize one of the primary ways we will be relating is by caring for our bodies. I have chronic lymphatic leukemia, which has not been treated yet. My body is doing great with it, but it is getting to the point where it is tired. Michael has slow-growing prostate cancer. How tender I feel about his body has changed from the sexuality at the beginning of our marriage to something else.

"We have to face the inevitability that it doesn't get much better. We are now talking about caretaking for each other. We say things like, 'Don't fall. Don't hurt yourself.' I want to care for myself so I don't have to be taken care of by him. There is a great tenderness to that and the anxiety of not knowing. I am not taking our health for granted as before. A couple of years ago, I slipped and fell in the bathroom and went to the emergency room. I lived through it because of his caretaking. I realized that this is not just about me anymore, but seeing how my health influences his day if I am debilitated. It was an experience of our interdependence."

Michael continued, "I'm finding the line between respecting this reality but not letting it make decisions for me. I don't want to make the fear of being hurt so intense that I don't enjoy life or do something I care about now. If something drastic happens to Eileen or me, I will gladly accept that as my next purpose in life. If that causes me to not ski as hard or much, that is fine and wonderful. This is part of our life together. On my bucket list is the desire to helicopter ski, which is not something Eileen could do now so I will do it by myself."

Physical challenges also take a toll on their sex lives. The Heatons name some realities that are often not discussed but were noted by a number of these couples. "The sexual part of your relationship takes a different place," Eileen said. "With all of the changes happening in our bodies, we feel this loss, which I am sorry about, but I can't be sexier than I feel. Sex has been less frequent but more important. I need to be physically connected, but it is not about sex. This feels like a loss, and I mourn it, yet, it is replaced with something else. It has taken some awareness and attention to start redefining it. This is a loss of what was once yummy. Something else that is more emotional, more spiritual, has taken its place, and it is a real change."

As elder couples renegotiate and help each other with changes in their physical bodies, this often leads to discerning whether they are living in the right home and environment. Michael and Eileen executed a significant change in their housing. They bought a condominium along the Deschutes River.

Eileen explained. "We both love gardening, but it is very time-consuming. We bought this place where we aren't tempted to garden anymore. It was a conscious decision, for we knew we were harming our bodies. It was a mindful choice to say, 'No more.' I worked as the choir director at First Presbyterian Church for eight years. I loved it, every moment of it. I loved being a conductor, as I had never done it before. And, yet, I was done with it. I knew, 'I love this, and I need to stop.'"

Michael noted, "I am laughing about the landscaping, for I am now board chair of our association here. I can plant a few bushes because I want to, but I don't have to do it. I try to decide if an activity is still enjoyable, and if so, I will do it. We sold off two rental projects. I managed them. When I realized I was looking for outside authority, I put them on the market in two weeks. As the eldest of five, I was given too much responsibility, too young. Eileen was right. Now at sixty-nine, I can divest this sense of responsibility. I don't need to carry it anymore. I would make four lunches for my siblings and cook oatmeal they hated. I don't need to keep carrying them."

We sensed that Michael and Eileen would share insights into the forgiveness process after all of the ups and downs of their lives and such an impressive commitment to their ongoing inner work and growth. We weren't disappointed.

Michael began, "Forgiveness is essential, and I am a novice at it, which goes back to my childhood. When things were volatile with the alcoholism in my family, I learned to duck for cover and wait for things to blow over. My main intention was for things to be okay and not to bring up the incident again. I still struggle with the anger I experienced from my father. I default to, 'Eileen is smiling, so everything is okay.' It has been hard for me to learn how to work things through. I get lost, and 'I am sorry' sounds trite. I have learned to say it, but I don't believe it myself, so it is hard to expect Eileen to believe me."

Eileen added, "I have a critical voice in my head, like my superego running crazy. I am so willing to accommodate being hurt. My primary need for forgiveness has been towards myself, which makes it possible to send the mercy of softening. 'I am sorry' pops out too easily. The idea of forgiveness directed towards Michael makes me think, 'Who am I to forgive him, for he is just doing his life?' But the idea of mercy includes an understanding that things didn't work out. This is a bad moment. Forgiveness has something in it about the other person having something on you. When in a place of comradery and compassion, we don't need to extend forgiveness, but mercy."

Eileen's insight about forgiveness struck us as original, noting that when you demand forgiveness from another, you place yourself in a one-up position over them and even play the victim. Mercy implies a drawing upon spiritual sources amid the struggles.

As our time with Michael and Eileen ended, we learned of some of their plans for the future, including exciting international travel and seeking treatment for their health issues. Michael was researching various options for his prostate cancer treatment, and Eileen acknowledged that soon her chronic lymphoma was going to need more care.

As they gradually begin to cut back on their work, they consider this a shift into a time to discover life beyond a focus on work and a time for deepening spiritually. From Michael's men's studies, he taught us about the four stages of life from Hinduism: The Student Stage is defined as preparing for success later in life, learning, studying, and obedience to a teacher. The Householder Stage includes marriage, work, and sustaining one's family. The Forest Dweller Stage occurs when the family duties have been fulfilled, and one withdraws from the fray. The Renunciation Stage occurs when, having fulfilled all prior obligations, one is free to devote one's life entirely to spiritual growth. Perhaps there is a natural renunciate stage awaiting us when one is widowed, or when age strips us of our capacity to live independently in our homes full of a lifetime of collected treasures. Age creates a built-in monastery at the threshold of our departure from this world.

Throughout our interviews, we noticed that most of the couples still cared about their callings and contributions, but more from the perspective of the Forest Dweller. They spend time reviewing their lives and questioning how best to use their limited remaining time and energy.

Eileen shared, "The thread for me is to live out whatever the Divine piece is within me and get out of the way of that. The ego grabs it and feels it has to push. I am working on that. Then there is further refinement, for I don't have the energy to teach forty-five hours a week. In the eldering process, how do I answer that call? As a spiritual director, I am trying to do less. There is a great deal to do, and I have never understood retirement. Why retire when we are at our wisest, smartest, and when we have incredible lived experience? I am not done but am phasing it out."

Elders become pickier about what they commit to and tend to commit to less.

Michael noted, "It is different because we are not both going at something twelve to fourteen hours a day. This started changing for me when we ended the full-time consultant gig. It felt like a glass wall I had pressed against, and then the wall came down. I support Eileen in the reduction of her teaching load. We don't need the money. I still have a couple of clients, and we work and prepare together for these clients. That helps us redefine what is happening between us."

When we no longer need to make money, it clarifies why we work. Not everyone can afford to retire, yet in these interviews, most people were working because they were called to do so, not to earn a living. There is great freedom in that. And often, great meaning as well.

These dear "Forest Dwellers" living along the Deschutes River Trail in the high desert of Central Oregon continue to creatively pivot and reinvent themselves, their lives anchored in deep respect, integrity, and capacity to work through life's many stages, side by side, in the spirit of mercy and grace.

The quality of mercy is not strained;
It droppeth as the gentle rain from heaven
Upon the place beneath: it is twice blest,
It blesseth him that gives and him that takes:
'Tis mightiest in the mightiest; it becomes
The thronèd monarch better than his crown.

WILLIAM SHAKESPEARE

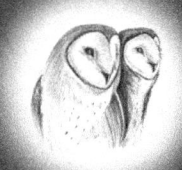

Blessed is the couple who
offers beneficial presence
across the generations, for they
shall leave a legacy of love.

BLESSED IS THE COUPLE WHO
Offers Beneficial Presence Across the Generations

INTRODUCING
RUTH SHAGOURY & JIM WHITNEY

WHEN JAY AND I were first inspired to interview couples, neither of us had a clue about how to begin. We had never operated a camera nor filmed people in an interview format, while Ruth and Jim had done both professionally. While visiting them in Portland over a weekend, we asked Jim for his advice on what equipment to purchase, and he said, "Oh, you can have my camera and stand. I no longer need them." He was retiring his videography work for good. Then Jim gave us a lifetime guarantee to help us learn how to use the equipment and finesse our way through the interviews, knowing full well the depth of our ineptitude when it comes to technology. (This later entailed taking our panicked calls from various locations across the country when we experienced breakdowns, and he dealt with our clueless blundering.) Ruth jumped in with her research background and her "heart of a mentor" for supporting others in their creative endeavors.

During that visit, Jim and Ruth spontaneously let us try out the camera and ask questions of them, which became our very first impromptu interview. It was a magical weekend, yet not unlike most of our time spent with them. Because the interview happened spontaneously, we ironically didn't spend as much time with them as the other couples in the project, yet our long-term, thirty-year friendship helped us fill in the gaps.

Jim and Ruth are transplants from New England, having met each other at the University of New Hampshire when they worked together, initially with Ruth serving as a research assistant for Jim. Jim explained, "I thought this assistant was pretty cool." They started seeing each other.

Ruth and Jim named many qualities that serve as a foundation for their compatibility: a strong work ethic, appreciation for each other's depth of intelligence, love of music, and easy communication. Ruth said to Jim, "You have a really good sense of humor, can be playful, are a genius, and are kind to me. I appreciate that. I used to feel you should tell me more that you love me. But I learned that you show me. I keep track. The kindest thing you ever did for me was when I was teaching at Lewis & Clark and getting home at 9 p.m. One time when I came in the front door, you had put my flannel cowgirl PJs in the dryer, made soup, sat me down, and took care of me. Who would think of putting PJs in the dryer to make them fluffy and warm? When I get agitated with you, Jim, I remember your kindnesses." What a great idea, keeping track of the kind things we do for each other, rather than hoarding up resentments and complaints.

Jim worked as an engineer, photographer, videographer, and all-around problem-solver. Ruth dedicated her career to teaching, writing, and researching, with a particular interest in how children and second language learners make sense of the world through speaking, writing, and art. When Ruth conducted interviews with children for her research, Jim filmed them. They helped each other often during their work lives.

Jay and I stayed with Jim and Ruth frequently after moving from Portland, Oregon, where we had worked with Ruth for thirteen years at Lewis & Clark College's graduate school, to Bend, a three-hour drive over the Cascade Mountains. They would also visit us and hike the trails along the Deschutes River near our home. These weekends together allowed for many shared meals and soul-satisfying conversations, the kind that could unfold over long mornings of sipping coffee in our PJs.

When you visit their home in Southeast Portland, it's not unusual for the doorbell to ring with a neighbor child hoping to go down into the basement to peruse the wall of children's books (and take one home), books collected over many years of devotion to teaching literacy. Ruth writes a *Lit for Kids* blog with her daughter, Meghan Rose, recommending current books to parents. Meg, a parent of twins who works in the internet start-up industry in Los Angeles, describes herself as an avid and ferocious reader. "The fruit doesn't fall far from the tree."

Ruth and Jim know how to play and practice the power of tomfoolery—something we noticed in other couples as well, which is why we felt it important to name it as a beatitude. The fireplace mantle displays "toys with attitude" gifted from friends, like a Ruth Ginsberg action figure or *Farts Around the World*, a book Jim proudly exhibits (with sound effects and all), a result of an ongoing fart joke he is running with the twins. As Martin Buber famously opined, "Play is the exultation of the possible." Whether they're talking with us, friends. or family, conversations are rich with new recipes, funny stories, and thoughts about emerging research on a myriad of subjects, including rants and outrage about politics, technological innovations, the latest Netflix series, struggles with family, health, and the challenges of aging. Jay and I always leave inspired and refreshed, like attending a stimulating university class.

Ruth's creativity and risk-taking are original, relational, and boundless. When teaching, she wouldn't ask students to write a report on a favorite author. Instead, she held tea parties and invited the students to roleplay authors, including dressing up as the persona of the writer. When she wanted to understand the lives of the graduate students, she followed one around for a day, then wrote about it. She convinced other faculty to do the same. When exploring the nature of creativity, she asked the students to bring in a snack based on the prompt, "What would creativity eat?" Ruth literally embodies creativity.

A lasting image we have of Ruth was when she was honored for receiving the Mary Stuart Rogers Professor of Education Endowed Chair at Lewis & Clark College for her outstanding record of teaching and publishing. When invited to march at the head of the line at graduation that year, she showed up with cowgirl boots displayed under her medieval black robe. (Ruth loves props and all things cowgirl.) Originality touches everything she approaches, including regular tasks in life, and her relationship with Jim. Creativity is the hallmark of their presence. When we find ourselves in the same room with them, it crackles with wicked humor.

Now, in retirement, Ruth and Jim have adjusted to stepping back from the intense focus on their work lives, embracing the new freedom retirement offers, and allowing themselves to enjoy the available time and space to live differently. Jim said, "I am still pretty focused. That didn't go away. Time has changed. Things have stretched out very nicely. That will never change. I am slower." Jim is methodical and thoughtful about what he commits to doing. The more spacious time in retirement affords him his natural style of taking time for his projects until he can get them where he wants them.

Ruth noted, "Jim, you still have plenty of projects. People call on you for help, and you are there. Now you have time for them. You fix computers and paint the stairs at your son's home. You set up a new TV for a widowed friend." Jim is skilled at what he sets his mind to learning and doing, capable of mastering complex technology, then generously offering his gifts to his friends and neighbors.

Ruth continued, "I am a planner and scheduler. I go to yoga every day. Yoga has become a central part of my life so that I can learn to relax and focus, and see my body get stronger, even though older. I thought I could just stay the same in my yoga practice, but I am still improving. It feels really good. I have no desire to teach it. I just like being a serious practitioner of yoga and understanding how my body works."

Many retirees report missing the structure that the workplace provided. Teachers miss the cycles of beginnings and endings, graduations, and summer breaks. Many find it valuable and necessary to create routines to frame their days in retirement.

"I was always focused on my identity as a teacher and writer," Ruth said. "Now, I see myself on vacation. I've worked since I was fifteen. Now I am grateful to read and walk and draw. I am savoring that my life is like a big vacation."

Ruth's dramatic step back from a life of intense dedication to her work brings to mind insights about aging from the work of Dr. Robert Johnson, a renowned Jungian therapist. In his book *Living Your Unlived Life*, Johnson notes that the way forward at this stage of life is not about repeating what we have done, but reclaiming the lost or neglected parts of ourselves that went underground, ignored, and underserved during the arduous, middle years of career and family. In his words, "By midlife your identity is the institutionalization of your past... In the second half of life we are called to live everything that we truly are, to achieve greater wholeness."[1]

Ruth added, "Because I am branching out in new ways, I am not an expert, especially in the things my kids are doing. By my example, I am an elder. Younger folks, we like to help them out, and sometimes serve as substitute grandparents. We see it as a gift to us. We deeply enjoy it. I was a teacher for so long. Now, I would rather be a learner, a beginner, and on vacation in many ways. I don't feel like an elder."

Jim, who loves children, noted, "The cool thing we experience with young friends is that in some ways we are in the role of adopted grandparents, or in the case of a young mother of a kid we spend time with, we are almost like an adopted parent. We are fairy godparents passing on wisdom." They delight in supporting a little girl named Vivian, whose mother is undergoing cancer treatment, inviting her for regular playdates, hosting tea parties, art projects, and ongoing fairy garden construction with her.

Ruth and Jim's twin grandchildren are their highest priority. Molly and Jacob visit every summer for two weeks, or during school breaks. Exciting family vacations with the twins include going to places like dude ranches, the Painted Hills of Oregon, or numerous city outings to science museums and hotel swimming pools. When apart, regular Zoom calls occur where they play games together, read and discuss books, or watch movies, bridging the distance between Los Angeles and Portland. Now that the twins are in their teens, Ruth and Jim stay near them in LA during their school vacations and work around Molly's Shakespeare Club meetings or her cooking show productions and Jacob's fencing practice. As you can imagine, Molly and Jacob adore them.

Jim and Ruth's relationships with young people remind us of a concept about eldering Jay picked up while teaching religious art history in Germany. He learned there is a phrase for the connection young people have in friendships with their elders, "Jugend und ältesten, austausch zwischen," meaning the intense, beneficial exchange between youth and elders, an expression that recognizes the energy transference from one generation to the other. It goes both ways, benefiting the young and the old alike. The elder offers a capacity to listen deeply and witness the young person's emerging gifts and interests, which often the parents are too busy and preoccupied to give. A space is created for refuge from their age-group pressures.

It's not only the twins that fill their lives with family time. Ruth has three brothers, and one sister who died from cancer, while Jim has a sister living in Florida. Ruth noted, "We are also closer to other family members, our nieces and nephews. Now that our parents have passed and we have retired, we can spread it out and visit Colorado and Maine to see the next generation. We Skype with them and get so much out of it. This is an extension of when we all had kids, and we saw each other in New England at our lake cabin. Now we get to know them as individuals, not just a big family."

With medical care what it is these days, extending life with various medications and surgeries, many people of our generation are approaching retirement with our parents still living. We are old people taking care of even older people. By the time of this interview, their parents had died after a very long decade of slow decline. Jim and Ruth navigated ten years when all four of their parents were diminished with various forms of dementia. Ruth's dad lived to age ninety-seven, and her mom, dying three months after he passed, at ninety-six. Jim's mom died at eighty-eight years old, while his dad lived to ninety.

Over the years, we heard their stories and witnessed their numerous trips to New Hampshire to arrange care, coordinate with their siblings, meet with lawyers, and spend time with their parents. They returned with hilarious yarns, chagrinned, drained, and humbled, yet their steadfast commitment to tend their parents generously and compassionately never wavered. Every time Ruth took a well-deserved sabbatical, a crisis would occur with her parents, and she spent many of those sabbatical months scrambling to help them. When Jim retired, he immediately faced managing his parents' finances, physical challenges, and estate, a time-consuming, demanding job. Handling repairs for their aging rural home from a distance on the opposite coast was especially trying. He eventually hired live-in help when his dad began slowly losing his executive powers.

Jim and Ruth embraced supporting their parents as education for facing this stage themselves. Ruth said, "It brought Jim and me closer instead of further apart. Both of our parents were failing at the same time. One parent would struggle, and we took turns focusing on them. Usually, it wasn't all of them at the same time. We knew what the other was going through. We did experience dissonance and felt frustrated when they were making our lives hard while also caring about them and not wanting them to die.

It is wonderful to have a partner who understands. It also teaches us what we do and don't want our relationship to be as we get older.

"One time my parents were playing cards and started laughing, realizing they weren't playing the same game. There was lots of laughter, for dementia has funny elements to it. They became very sweet and forgave each other for earlier foibles."

Jim chimed in, "Later you will understand when you watch Ruth and I have parallel conversations. I agree with Ruth. It was an amazing window for considering a point I hadn't thought of before when we get old. We talk about what we can do better when we get there and not put our family members through what we went through. It was a big lesson, one we are still working on. What do we want to do differently? I want to be quicker and more aggressive about shedding stuff, and lightening up what we accumulated. It is hard to plan for the moment when you lose the capacity to function, for it can be such a slow slide. I am not prepared for how to deal with that one yet."

Jim's comments reminded me of a conversation I attempted with my parents as they turned eighty. They were still living in the home they built in 1950, still driving, and living the life they always had known, but slowing down. Dad was having strokes and other health problems. When I asked my mom what her plans were for their next steps, she said, "We are taking it a day at a time." It was an honest answer. While baffled at the time, now in my 70s, I understand. You don't know what is ahead, how you will exit this life, or what you will need next. Regardless, it is worth reflecting on when we are still healthy and taking steps as best we can to prepare so that making decisions is easier for our families.

Ruth described their approach to such steps. "We were teaching our kids along the way. I was aware of my future care, and I kept saying, 'We want Grandpa well-cared for. This is his money. They wouldn't be looking for the cheapest option if they could do this themselves.' That is what you do for your kids; you model these things. We are there for our parents the way they were there for us when we were young. I don't want them to cater to us, but the generations are important to each other. We didn't want any regrets when they died. What we gave up to visit them, including the financial strain and vacations for our pleasure, wasn't important. We did the best we could. We talked about this with each of our kids at the time. We hired a good estate lawyer. We meet every few years, and she wanted to meet our kids. Someday, when they come to settle our estate, they will have a relationship with her. It doesn't seem real yet."

Jim added, "Our kids don't want to talk about that yet. It was nothing I thought about until Dad's financial advisor said it was time to take it over for him. I was shocked and asked, 'For what?' They weren't doing very well, so I did it. It was pretty amazing."

When we asked the couples in our interviews what their greatest fear about aging was, they all said they feared dementia, Alzheimer's disease, or something to that effect, and becoming a burden on others. In that vein, Ruth shared the following piece of writing, where she captures the love, grief, and mystery we undergo when we love people who are no longer entirely with us, whom we lose a piece of, an inch at a time. Jim's support, insight, and sensitivity are precisely what we can do for one another, side by side, when we sit with our grief and loss.

MY MOTHER'S HANDS[2]

My mother's hands felt papery-dry as I began to rub lotion into them. Her joints and knuckles were large and knobby and made her thin wrists and fingers look gnarled. With long, tender strokes, I massaged the lavender oil into each finger, caressing her skin and holding the mental image of pouring my love through our hands as they touched, hoping she could sense my feelings for her.

She was so distant now as she stared vaguely out of sunken, pale blue eyes. But as I massaged her hands and arms, she responded with a rare energy.

"Oh," she sighed. "That feels so good. You can't know how good that feels." Her eyes turned to me and seemed to hold more light. I whispered, "I'm so glad," as I held her warm hand in mine. "I wish I could do it for you," she continued, squeezing my hand and sending a warm surge through my body. I held a strong image of her massaging my hands and legs with such tender care when I was tired as a child, or brushing the tangles out of my long hair. I wanted to hold on to the moment, that vital connection between us I had not felt for over a year. "Where do you live now?' she asked, meeting my eyes. "I'm still in Portland, Oregon—a long trip from New Hampshire..." Her eyes lit up. "My daughter lives in Portland!" "Yes, it's me! It's Ruthie!" My eyes sought hers, pleading for recognition. "Oh, my daughter's name is Ruthie, too! She's a good girl. You'd like her."

I felt the tears coming to my eyes, as they do again as I remember. I had thought we were sharing a rare moment of clarity and recognition in the darkness of her dementia, that she knew it was me here with her. Later that evening, I told Jim the story of my afternoon, crying my despair, aching for a true connection again with my mother. To be known.

Now it was Jim who took my hand, warming it as he held it between his. "She does know you. She knows she has a daughter—and she's a good girl. She knows if people met her Ruthie, they'd like you." He paused. "She knows that—and I do, too."

These days, as she sinks deeper and deeper into confusion, I hold on to our time together that cold winter day—when I felt our bond—and know that in her way, she felt it, too.

Even though she didn't know who I was.

A lasting image we will always carry of Ruth and Jim is of two people holding hands, living side by side, nurturing the generations in both directions of their lives, creatively improvising, and enjoying the time they still have left together.

Be kind whenever possible. It is always possible.
HIS HOLINESS THE DALAI LAMA

Love takes off the masks that we fear we cannot live without and know we cannot live within. I use the word "love" here not merely in a personal sense but as a state of being, or a state of grace—not in the infantile American sense of being made happy but in the tough and universal sense of quest and daring and growth.

JAMES BALDWIN

CONCLUSION

Lessons from the Road to *Side by Side*

BY
JAY CASBON

AS THE *SIDE BY SIDE* project shifted to the writing phase, we immersed ourselves in transcribing eighty-four hours of recordings from the interviews. We knew, at some point, that we would also need to answer the questions: "How about your story as a couple? Where do you fit in all of this?" And, "What did you learn?"

Caryl and I found ourselves in a mild state of melancholy. It was sad to let go of the sweet thrills of the project's beginnings, such as deciding whom to interview, and developing our questions and format in a secluded, cozy cabin during a three-week artist residency at Playa, in the wild, isolated spaces of the Great Basin of Oregon. We felt nostalgic about the stimulating travel, visiting couples in their homes, and the powerful connections with them, times now fading in the rearview mirror. Finally, we reluctantly sold the Dharma Dog (our Winnebago) when we returned to Oregon. It would be impractical for our upcoming move to a new living situation in Santa Barbara. We felt dejected driving away from the sales lot, like abandoning a loyal old hound dog at the Humane Society. The journey now called us inward, and time demanded we settle down in one place to write.

In the spirit of transparency, before summarizing our findings from the interviews, we want to describe the ordeal we experienced with our own relationship. This is no hero/ego story; it is our soul story.

Married twenty years, we encountered an alchemy of extraordinary circumstances during the course of this project: retirement, health problems, leaving Oregon to move to California, the impact and isolation from the COVID-19 pandemic, and the backdrop of political unrest, drought, and wildfires destroying our sacred forests in the West. Now, as we conclude this book, we confront multiple threats of war, out-of-control inflation, and a breakdown of civility, democracy, and public discourse. Our generation is aging in remarkable times, just like the times in which we came of age. The losses and threats increase daily, both individually and collectively.

Several therapist friends cautioned, "If you start researching the lives of couples, all of your issues will soon be in your faces." Our astrologer, Carol Ferris, alerted us that our partnership was heading into a phase of renegotiating all terms established in the past. We didn't really know what she meant at the time, but looking back, we see what her warning foretold.

While I was traveling cross-country for a month with my sons and brother in the fall of 2021, Caryl became highly anxious, feeling cut off from me and fearful I was leaving her. As soon as I returned, we agreed, "We need help." We didn't really know what was wrong. Still, we experienced painful symptoms: a growing distance from each other, both of us "spring-loaded" in reactive, angry, defensive positions, feeling sad, lonely, frustrated with ourselves, and very disappointed in our marriage. We acknowledged that our relationship appeared way too similar to our parents' post-WWII-1950s relationships.

Our energy signature was dimmed, at best. We felt out of integrity doing this project, as we asked, "How in the world can we go public with this book when we are such a mess?" We knew we were sitting on a taxing but vital opportunity to grow. As soon as we acknowledged our problems, assistance began to appear.

We were introduced to the groundbreaking work of Dr. Terry Real, who, based on 45 years of practice as a couple's therapist, pointed out the obvious: we live in a society that doesn't really value relationships, with many of us "relationally unfit" and adrift. We immediately enrolled in several of his programs and studied his books and videos.[1] Briefly, we learned that our generation's relationships, while formed in the heady era of the human potential and women's liberation movements, are still largely stuck in the past, following the patriarchal, gender-role-defined patterns modeled by our parents. Even more daunting, Real claims that we marry our unfinished business from our family of origin experiences. In fact, we are drawn to just the person who will put this "business" in our faces so we can heal, not only ourselves, but these ancestral patterns. It is actually the path to growth; whom you marry becomes the doorway to your development. Yikes. Who signed up for this?

In therapy, I began to address how Caryl hooks my unconscious "adaptive child" reactions formed in my relationship with my mother, who was deeply wounded from her own abusive childhood. Mom's parenting was scattered and chaotic. She was often not present and physically neglectful at times. With Caryl, I developed a "take charge" approach, learned to hide my feelings and vulnerability, even from myself, focused on work and intellectual pursuits, and tried to control our relationship as much as possible. Because our conflicts made these patterns visible, I can now work with them in the open and catch the projection of my mother issues onto Caryl, and know when my adaptive child has taken over. Coincidentally, I also remind Caryl of her mother, who was very judgmental, unpredictable, controlling, emotionally distant, and withdrawn at times, leaving her feeling abandoned, untrusting, and insecure. When coming from this wounded child (which thankfully isn't all the time), she is hypersensitive, defensive, often doesn't trust me, and thinks I don't love her. We aren't alone. Many couples in the interviews share how their relationships have brought them to their shadow work. For us, part of the "sacred art of relationship" is addressing these issues and undergoing the humbling task of shadow work.

With the grace of an outstanding therapist, we continue to learn, make changes, and accept that our partnership is a work in slow-motion progress, revealing insights and opportunities one session at a time. It's one thing to bring these shadows out into the open, but another thing to drop old patterns. Change takes time. Like any living organism, our relationship is dynamic, evolving, and still emerging into new dimensions. We can't relax, nor do we take our progress for granted. We feel so much better, transformed and transforming, yet get discouraged at times when we "step in it" and act out of our old patterns. At those times, we try to practice mercy, kindness, and extend grace.

Finally, during this project, we decided to cease regularly drinking alcohol, our habituated ritual of numbing out and stuffing our feelings by consuming fine wines every night. We recently embraced a plant-based diet in order to do less harm to the planet and our aging bodies. We are, truly, a work in progress. This is our soul story, for which we thank the *Side by Side* project and the couples involved.

From the years of struggling and wrestling with our marriage (and past relationship failures as well) and finally facing some of our deeper frailties described above, I am experiencing what I have come to think of as "good exhaustion." When we work out in the gym, we feel "good exhaustion" from pushing our muscles, and even though it hurts, we get stronger. While a part of me wanted to stay home on the couch and avoid this heavy emotional lifting with Caryl, I earned the satisfaction and growth from wrestling with painful, unresolved issues. I got tired and, at times, wanted to quit. I always drove myself hard in my career and expected it would be difficult, but I didn't know that intimate relationships were so much work. We found that our spiritual covenant established in marriage, "in sickness and in health," sustained us through the storms. Many of the couples we interviewed noted that the key to their relationship health was directly connected to each in the relationship facing their shadow work.

As I considered how to summarize our findings, as a retired university professor, I recalled how my students counted on me to provide a syllabus for my courses, including objectives, central concepts, and what I expected them to learn. Well, in this case, I offer the syllabus in reverse order, humbly acknowledging that you have hopefully found your own conclusions and meaning in the narratives.

Below is a list of characteristics, insights, and realities many of these aging couples of our generation share in common—a community zeitgeist of sorts, out of which glimpses of the larger story may appear.

1. **Partners with Spirit** If there is one quality the *Side by Side* couples share in common, it is best

described as being spiritual seekers. This generation came of age as the mysteries of many world faith traditions—including the bodies of esoteric knowledge from astrology, the occult, and indigenous spiritual wisdom—suddenly opened up to us through teachers, programs, the internet, books, podcasts, cult movements, pilgrimages, and retreats. Those who stayed with their faith traditions worked to reform them and were outspoken about the egregious abuses of religion. Most of these couples don't attend church, and none of their children do. Regardless of their paths, they acknowledge the Divine's central role as the common ground at the core of their relationship. Contemplative in nature, many pray and/or meditate together and draw on spiritual guidance for discernment when in trouble or in need of direction. With serious conflict, loss, or challenge, they turn to Spirit. In other words, the Divine is a partner and presence in their marriages. The covenant of marriage supports them in staying together through difficult times.

2. **The Gift of Mutuality** Mutuality is the capacity to care about the other's well-being, needs, and preferences as much as our own. Because couples live and breathe together in a communal biosphere, their welfare is intimately interconnected. While each person stands confident in their differentiation, they sometimes strive to soften the "I" to embrace the "we" when practicing mutuality.

3. **Welcoming the Stranger** Couples become strangers to one another because people change and evolve. It can be challenging to stay alert to the shifting passions,

interests, and creative expressions in one another. While it can threaten stasis, healthy couples welcome this "strangeness" as a sign of new life. They understand that change brings fresh waters to the well of the marriage. They value, make room for, and greet the growing edges in one another.

4. **The Practice of Kindness & Service**   The heart for kindness and service is fundamental in relationships. So essential are the many small acts of kindness, they become the very glue of an affectionate marriage. When kindness becomes muted or lost, the marriage feels ragged and unsafe. As health problems ensue with aging, some couples named the need to be more in service to one another, volunteering less in the community, and instead devoting themselves to assisting one another.

5. **Wisdom & Beneficial Presence**   No one in this project would claim themselves as wise or even an elder, yet throughout the interviews, their beneficial presence and wisdom were evident. While elusive to describe, we noticed a few patterns in the wisdom that emanates from these elders. Wisdom increases over time in a person who is committed to their own interiority and contemplative practices, meaningful work, and service. Innately humble, wisdom acknowledges the poverty of the ego and emerges out of the deeper qualities of the soul, rooted in the Source. Inherently resilient, wisdom understands how to use suffering for growth and supports others in doing so as well. Wisdom knows one can't take on the pain for another, nor possibly understand what they need, but influences others with quiet listening, grounded presence, example, and care. Wisdom surrenders outcomes to the Divine and knows

it is not for us to judge. Wisdom lives in deep time, honoring wholeness and the cycles of birth, death, and resurrection.

6. **Aging as a Team Sport**   Partnerships develop relational fitness when they team up and undertake whatever challenges arise, drawing on their combined resources. *Side by Side* couples often named how they are "stronger together" as they tackle the trials of life and aging, with each person contributing their differing gifts to the situation. "We have each other's back" is often expressed as a statement of fact.

7. **Seeking Help**   One of the greatest gifts we can give each other is to seek counseling when up against destructive patterns. Whether they be addictions, unconscious childhood wounds, trauma, unattended grief, or breakdowns in intimacy, these can be times when we sadly inflict violence on the one we love most. It is the nature of relationships to act out our wounds with each other, and those wounds can, with an honest partner, be mirrored back to us. It is up to the couple to take on these concerns and seek outside help, for the rewards of healing are immense. Richard Rohr is often cited for saying pain that is not transformed is pain that is transmitted. Problems that go untended turn into unhealthy symptoms that grow larger and more hurtful over time.

8. **The Dance of Gender Roles**   In terms of division of labor, gender role issues were reported as easily managed. However, the gender role modeling from our parents was not easily overcome. While aspiring to be intimate soul mates and companions, the realities

of gender role patterns persist in this generation's committed relationships, especially for the men, who discussed the limits of their masculine programming. For the men, hard work and providing for the family were emphasized, at the cost of being cut off from their feelings, their partners, and their children. In general, their fathers haunt them, and there is compunction about their lives. For the women, many still struggle with focusing on caring for others over self-care and establishing an equal footing in their relationships.

9. **Parenting Never Ends**   For couples with children, stepchildren included, parenting never stops. Adult children still need attention, affection, and support. In fact, at this time of life, these relationships are of the highest priority. As their adult children face their destinies, often fraught with divorces, job losses, financial difficulties, addictions, etc., we can no longer shield them from the pain of life as when they were babies. As elders, we can offer them the gifts of listening, witnessing, and supporting their decisions and life directions. We celebrate their achievements and adore their children. If we hold clear boundaries and avoid the traps of telling them what to do or judging them, the rewards are immense. Finally, our couples noted that if their relationships with their children were neglected or harmed earlier in life, this is a time for healing, truth-telling, forgiveness, and reconciliation.

10. **The Loss of the World as We Knew It**   Just as this generation shocked, alienated, and distanced from parents as they approached adulthood in "The Age of Aquarius," and "Don't trust anyone over 30," we now experience a growing generation gap with our adult

children's realities. Baby boomers, ironically, now bear the brunt of ageism, ridiculed and blamed in the media for the mounting global problems and shabby leadership. So much has changed; our mid-century beginnings appear remote at best. As we observe the dimming of the cultural memories, rock stars, music, historical markers, and achievements that define our generation, there is a sense of displacement from a world moving forward without us. We have become *strangers in a strange land*, deeply concerned about the future of our children.

11. **Freedom from Function**   An exhilarating sense of "freedom from function" was highlighted by the *Side by Side* couples. No longer controlled by the needs of the first half of life, these couples celebrated their liberation. Mostly free from the necessities of earning a living, professionally proving oneself, raising a family, etc., there are fresh opportunities to explore their unlived lives, know themselves more deeply, discern emerging priorities, play, and define how to be in service and use their time.

12. **Passion, Meaning & Purpose**   While the stereotype of aging couples is one of the elders parked in rocking chairs on the front porch, slowly fading from public view, we did not find this at all. These couples are active, often trying out new skills. Many dedicate themselves to creative endeavors like painting or writing books, memoirs, and plays. Others commit to social activism, volunteering, or deepening intellectual pursuits. Some serve as consultants, thought partners, mentors, spiritual counselors, or in board leadership roles. They all offer a "ministry of presence" by aiding family members in need and building closer connections with

friends, neighbors, their children, and grandchildren. None of the couples mentioned being bored, but they did discuss the vital role of soul-directed discernment in establishing priorities. Discerning life direction is an inside job. The couples expressed impatience with things like committee work or anything that feels like a waste of time. They are intensely aware of the ticking clock and that their time left is finite.

13. **Financial Tending**   These couples pay attention to forging economic security as a way of caring for and protecting their legacies and their children's future. Investments, property, inheritances, and sometimes establishing a family trust are attended to. In second marriages, some had to learn to integrate fair treatment of their blended family. Others had to create plans for retirement, knowing their current finances as inadequate.

14. **The Power of Touch**   Physical intimacy maintains attunement and connection and is critical to the health of a relationship at any stage. With age, this need does not diminish; it changes. Every couple underlined the importance of enjoying physical contact with one another and some melancholy about how they once were together in younger bodies. Humor was never far off when discussing aging bodies and intimacy.

15. **Befriending Uncertainty**   Difficult to plan for, aging together is full of uncertainty. There are many potential threats just waiting to befall a couple: physical and/or cognitive impairment, death of a partner, loss of friends to death and illness, or a sudden onset of diseases, such as a heart attack or cancer. These couples help each

other to pay gentle attention to their bodies, report they need more rest, and that they don't handle stress as well. Becoming savvy in the face of a new limit, *Side by Side* couples discussed supporting each other by drawing on the capacity to pivot, be of service to each other, and creatively adapt to changing conditions.

16. **Gifts from the Departed Ancestors**   Some of the best moments in the interviews happened when the couples explored the stories of their parents' deaths. Just as children constantly watch their parents in order to learn, our couples revealed how they were schooled in loss and death by witnessing their mothers and fathers age and die. These stories live close to their hearts as their parents continue to teach them from beyond the grave. Death doesn't end our relationships with our parents; many reported a continued connection with a father or mother, or grandparent, now in Spirit.

17. **Approaching Death**   No one in this project claimed to fear death. Some expressed playful curiosity about what might be on the other side of this life and viewed death as a continuation of their souls into Spirit, from life to more life. Many recounted mystical experiences while accompanying others in dying and view death as a "thin place," inextricably connected to birth, both natural and necessary. However, most noted that they fear dementia and being a burden on others as they approach the end of life, as well as dreading the thought of losing each other.

18. **Awe, Gratitude, and Hope**   In the process of interviewing these couples, many noted how thankful they are to have a partner at a time in life when so many are alone. They are in awe of and grateful for how rich

their lives have been and continue to be. They savor the slower pace of their lives and feel hopeful for what may lie ahead as they face the uncertainties of their future, side by side.

Finally, none of these couples would describe their marriages as "Happy Ever After." That would be an ego story. The soulful nature of relationships is far more complex, nuanced, and challenging than a fairy tale ending implies. A relationship is a safe harbor, yet one that sometimes tosses couples into the storms of the open seas. The soul story acknowledges the relationship struggles as vital to maturation. Perhaps "Happy After All" better captures the sacramental nature of relationships where partners must surrender their idealistic fantasy of the fairy tale nature of love; soften their defensive, reactive, "anti-relational programs"; and dance with differences. Sometimes it's a line dance, tango, or waltz. At others, it's a circle dance. There is no better dance we know of, all in all.

I hope that we can experience bliss. I want us to sense how big life is—how intense, joyful, painful, complicated, and beautiful our lives can be. Let us embrace everything. This can be our rescue as we navigate this last stretch of the river with its treacherous currents, quicksand, deep clear waters, and silver sunsets.

MARY PIPHER

*Our relationships live in the
space between us which is sacred . . .
All real living is meeting.*

MARTIN BUBER

Acknowledgments

FROM ITS INCEPTION, *Side by Side* has been communal in nature, inspired and guided by Spirit, and co-created with the couples interviewed for this book. They not only welcomed us into their relationships and homes but also patiently remained engaged throughout the following years, reading drafts of their chapters, answering questions, and offering suggestions.

While writing this book, grace appeared through the unearned, generous, and surprising offerings of many friends, but especially Jim Whitney and Ruth Shagoury, who were our dream partners from the get-go, egging us on and extravagantly offering their wisdom, expertise, and camera equipment, along with ongoing technical and creative encouragement.

We wish to thank Ellie Waterson and the PLAYA artist and writers residency center in Summer Lake, Oregon, where we enjoyed three weeks of isolation and privacy to incubate the questions that shaped the interviews. We thank our circle of friends in Bend, who generously tendered their interest and excitement for the project. We thank our housemate, Georgia Noble, who listened to the endless ups and downs throughout the isolating years of the pandemic, and beyond. We thank our therapist, Thery Jenkins, with the Family Therapy Institute of Santa Barbara, who showed us a way through a dark time in our relationship and continues to support us as we strive to embody the Beatitudes for Couples. We acknowledge the many influences of the Center for Courage & Renewal, for the Circle of Trust process and the network of soulful friends and colleagues who comprise many couples interviewed. We thank Parker and Sharon Palmer for hosting us on our journey and encouraging us in this project. We are indebted to Shelly Francis, who had the guts to gently tell us our first draft needed work and has liberally contributed her editing gifts over time. We are grateful to our church home and the leadership of Reverend Elizabeth Molitors and Reverend Sarah Dammann Thomas at Trinity Episcopal Church in Santa Barbara, California, who have been steadfast in supporting our work. And finally, we thank Maryellen Kelly, our dear friend, now with Spirit, who guides us and inspires us with her eternal presence, humor, and wisdom. **We are so grateful!**

APPENDIX I

Interview Questions for the *Side by Side* Project

THE INTERVIEWS OF each couple, approximately six hours long and conducted over several days, followed a structure based on the questions below. The questions target the three themes this book explores—relationships, spirituality, and aging—and were organized into six sections to gently explore this territory:

- PART I Coming Together & Staying Together
- PART II Seasons of Change & Challenge
- PART III Loss & Gains Through Life's Transitions
- PART IV Meaning & Purpose
- PART V Creating Sanctuary & Spiritual Sustenance
- PART VI Wisdom & Maturity

The intention behind using these questions was to create an opportunity for each couple to look deeply into their relationship history and practices, to be witnessed and honored for who they are as a couple, and consider their plans for this time of life, as well as for us to glean and share their wisdom as they reflected on where they are now as a couple. Each interview was filmed and recorded, and the couples received a copy to share with their children and family.

You are invited to use this interview process in a myriad of ways: in a retreat setting with other couples; in the privacy of your home, answering a question each day and sharing it with your partner; in friendship couples' circles, neighborhood groups, or with your children; and so on. Enjoy!

PART I: COMING TOGETHER & STAYING TOGETHER

1. What is the story of what brought you together? What keeps you together?
2. What foundational, core values did you share in your beginnings as a couple, and how (or have) those values changed over time?
3. When you committed to each other, what did love mean to you?
4. What does love mean to you now?
5. What has most tested your love?
6. What did you learn about love from your family of origin, and how has that impacted your relationship?
7. Tell a story about how your partner shows their love to you.
8. When do you feel most loved by your partner?
9. Would you share some stories about some of the highlights of your partnership?
10. What have been the greatest lessons in your relationship?
11. If you could design a tattoo for your partner that captures their spirit, what would it be, and where would you place it?

PART II: SEASONS OF CHANGE & CHALLENGE

1. What has been the biggest surprise for you at this stage of your relationship?
2. How have you witnessed your partner change over time? What has stayed the same?

3. How is aging impacting gender roles and sexuality issues in your relationship?
4. What would it look like to cooperate with your own aging?
5. Describe how your partner handles change. How are you alike and different in this area?
6. What do you imagine is most difficult about you that your partner needs to live with? In other words: What is it about me that is hard for them, that defies changing or fixing.
7. When going through challenges, how do you seek Spirit in the midst of them? Can you give an example?
8. What does restoration look like for you through your conflicts?
9. What have been the most important lessons you have learned from each other as a result of your conflicts, differences, and disagreements?
10. Describe your forgiveness process with each other. Can you give an example of it?
11. If you were each an animal, what would you be? (Name this for each other).

PART III: LOSS & GAINS THROUGH LIFE'S TRANSITIONS

1. What sort of losses (physical, mental, material, etc.) have you faced so far in relation to your aging? What sort of losses and challenges, if any, are you working with now?
2. Describe how you have worked together on these losses and how they impact your partnership. What kinds of adjustments are you making concerning these changes?
3. Tell the stories of your parents' (or other important people's) passing. What did you learn from them as they transitioned from this life?
4. What conversations about your own deaths are you having or not? What preparations, if any, have you pursued? What are your thoughts about "preparing" for your death?

5. How does your spirituality inform your understanding of death and your mortality?
6. At this stage of life, with death in the not-so-distant future, how does its presence impact your relationship with each other, with yourselves, with time?
7. What will be hard for you to leave behind when you die?
8. What do you fear most at this time about your aging?
9. If you could give your partner an object to take with them to the other side, what would it be? Something to pack in a final carry-on, so to speak.

PART IV: MEANING & PURPOSE

1. You often hear people, after someone dies in a ski accident, or mountain climbing, say, "At least they died doing what they loved." Name for your partner what it would look like if he or she died doing what they love.
2. If you could name it in three or four words, what captures the essence of your life's work up until now—what would those words be?
3. At this stage of life, what are you most passionate about? In other words, how do you define your calling, your dharma, or life purpose? How do you pursue your passions at this age? As individuals as well as a couple?
4. Are there "areas of interest" in terms of creativity that you are pursuing at this time, or hoping to pursue?
5. Where do you find risk-taking in your life, now that you aren't meeting challenges and risks constantly in your work world?
6. As a couple, what can you say "hell yes" to at this stage of your lives? Where are the places of shared meaning and depth?
7. What kind of discernment practices do you engage in as a couple, to determine your priorities in terms of how to spend your resources and energy?

8. Are there things in your life that are beginning to feel like a waste of time?
9. If you could throw a party for your spouse that is tailor-made to delight them, filled with what they love, whom they love, fun and games, and surprise guests (dead or alive), what would you create? (If your partner hates parties, modify this question to suit them.)

PART V: CREATING SANCTUARY & SPIRITUAL SUSTENANCE

1. Share your story of how you have pursued your spiritual lives, individually and together, over the course of your relationship.
2. How do you manage the "alone/together" balance in your relationship? How do you "protect one another's solitude?"
3. What mystical experiences, if any, have you undergone?
4. What does it mean to you to age together in Spirit?
5. What is your spiritual covenant as a couple?
6. How do you invite the Divine into your relationship?
7. How are you the same, and how are you different in the ways you seek to connect with the Creator?
8. How can you help or hinder each other's relationship with God?
9. If you could assign an animal guardian or protector, celestial being, archangel, wise soul, etc., to accompany your partner, what would it look like or be?

PART VI: WISDOM & MATURITY

1. What does maturity mean to you in this relationship?
2. What role does wisdom play in your relationship with each other?
3. What role does wisdom play in aging?

4. What dreams do you have for your relationship going forward?
5. What do you hope your legacy as a couple will be?
6. What wisdom do you have about relating to nurturing your adult children?
7. What do you hope your children and other loved ones will say about you when you are gone?
8. What have you learned from this interview process?
9. Is there anything we didn't ask that you would like to ask and answer to enhance this interview?

APPENDIX II

Touchstones for Couples' Group Work

FACILITATORS OF COURAGE & RENEWAL programs use these Touchstones to define clear boundaries in a Circle of Trust retreat, the kinds of boundaries that create trustworthy space for the soul. These Touchstones support any relationship, workplace, community, or other groups where we want to honor the integrity of the individual and build relational trust. Download a printable version at www.sidebysideaging.com.

EXTEND AND RECEIVE WELCOME.

People learn best in hospitable spaces. In this circle we support each other by giving and receiving hospitality, both to what comes up from within, as well as what is shared in the community.

**WHAT IS OFFERED IN THIS CIRCLE IS
BY INVITATION, NOT DEMAND.**

This is not a "share or die" event! During this meeting, do whatever your soul calls for, and know that you do it with our support. Your soul knows your needs better than we do.

**SPEAK YOUR TRUTH IN WAYS THAT RESPECT
THE TRUTH OF OTHER PEOPLE.**

Our views of reality may differ, but speaking one's truth in a circle of trust does not mean interpreting, correcting, or debating what others say. Speak from your center to the center of the circle, using "I" statements, trusting people to do their own sifting and winnowing.

NO FIXING, NO SAVING, NO ADVISING, AND NO CORRECTING EACH OTHER.

This is one of the hardest guidelines. But it is vital to welcoming the soul, and for making space for the inner teacher. When someone speaks in this gathering, we simply listen and receive their sharing with silent attention.

WHEN THE GOING GETS ROUGH, TURN TO WONDER.

If you feel judgmental, or defensive, ask yourself, "I wonder what brought her to this belief?" "I wonder what he's feeling right now?" "I wonder what my reaction teaches me about myself?" Set aside judgment to listen to others—and to yourself—more deeply.

ATTEND TO YOUR OWN INNER TEACHER.

We learn from others, of course. But as we explore stories, questions, and silence, we have a special opportunity to learn from within. So, pay close attention to your own reactions and responses, to your most important teacher.

OBSERVE DEEP CONFIDENTIALITY.

Nothing said in this meeting will ever be repeated to other people.

Adapted from the Circle of Trust® Touchstones of the Center for Courage & Renewal, founded by author/educator Parker J. Palmer. See www.couragerenewal.org/courage-renewal-approach/

[When aging] we do not need formulas or rigid models to follow; we need to be drawn into a common process of search that will suggest new ways of being.

MARY CATHERINE BATESON

READERS' GUIDE

Exploring the Stories & Themes in *Side by Side*

IN THE PROCESS of conducting the interviews with the *Side by Side* couples, without exception, each thanked us for the undivided attention we gave to their relationship. We followed the same format each time and spent at least six hours filming them as they answered the same questions (listed in appendix I). We then gifted them with a copy of the film so they could share it with their children if they wished or simply watch the interview and ponder what they had said.

We noticed how there are few places where couples are witnessed and cherished by others. Strangely, couples in committed relationships are often isolated and lack support and attention. In that spirit, we offer this Readers' Guide to assist you in engaging with your own soul stories by reflecting on your aging, spiritual life, relationship, and plans for this time of life. If you would like to invite other couples to read the book together and explore what it means to approach relationships as a "sacred art" and "age together in wisdom and love," as the title of the book invites you to consider, this Readers' Guide provides the structure for a small-group process.

Here we offer suggestions for how to organize an ongoing study group using the Circle of Trust approach, which is based on the work of author/educator Parker J. Palmer and the facilitators prepared by the Center for Courage & Renewal. Pair this guide with the Touchstones (in appendix II) to create a trustworthy space. For additional resources and guidance, go to the authors' website: www.sidebyside aging.com.

DESIGNING A *SIDE BY SIDE* COUPLES' GROUP

After thirty-five years of leading and teaching groups of all stripes, we've learned how essential it is for them to have clear leadership and boundaries so participants know how to listen, respond, and be together while avoiding some of the problems common to group life. Since the narratives in *Side by Side* model and invite vulnerable sharing, it is especially important that these "rules for engagement" be followed. This design, along with the Touchstones, creates the boundaries for how to be together to ensure respectful listening, safety, confidentiality, and honesty.

The Work Before the Work

If you are considering forming a group to explore the themes and ideas in *Side by Side*, please prepare yourselves first by taking the time to work through the program with your partner by both reading the book and answering the questions in this guide. It is the best and only way to make ready for leading this work. In the process, you will become familiar with the themes, try out some of the practices, and also discern who you think is appropriate to invite to your group. This level of depth inner work is not for everyone.

Leadership

We recommend one person or a two-person team/couple lead a *Side by Side* Couples' Group and that the leaders have a background in working with small groups. Do not pass the leadership around. The leader's role is to keep time, schedule sessions, send out reminders of the meetings, initiate and participate in the sharing, and gently guide the group back to the process if it goes off track.

Group Size

The ideal size of a group is between six to twelve members (i.e., three to six couples). The larger the group, the more likely you will need to divide it into smaller units to ensure adequate time for sharing. In most cases, since this is for couples, you will often spend time in dyads or groups of four. Keep in mind that the larger the group, the more leadership, skill, and coordination will be required. We recommend you start small.

Frequency & Timing of the Meetings

In addition to the introductory material, there are thirteen chapters, one for each couple's story, which focuses on one beatitude, as well as other themes. It is, of course, up to the group to choose how many chapters to address and how long and frequently you wish to convene. You could begin with a few sessions, or schedule a group to meet monthly or more often and work through the entire book. If you choose to address only one or two chapters in the collection, a single meeting will suffice. The chapters can be read in any order. If you are offering a group in a church or community setting, it is a good idea to first present an introductory session and then invite the couples to discern whether they wish to continue. In this manner, people often self-select, and this can save frustration for all concerned. No one should be coerced to participate.

Whom to Invite

The purpose of this group is to create conversations that address the intersection between growing older together, the spiritual dimensions of aging, and making the most of the last chapter of life. As you invite others into this exploration, you can start small by inviting two to three other couples you know and consider appropriate—call this your pilot group. When the word gets out about what you are doing and others begin to show interest, you can expand from there. If you are offering a group in your church or a nonprofit organization, consult with the leadership team regarding who may be right for your group or who may not.

We want to acknowledge that this program calls forth a deep level of openness. Both people in a relationship must be willing to participate and not feel coerced. Some men of this generation are not familiar with inner work and see vulnerability as unsafe or even unmanly and may opt out for that reason. Some people are simply too private and don't want to expose their relationships to others. Some experience with inner work is helpful. Most relationships are dynamic, living entities that experience varying degrees of conflict and tension. If couples are willing to and capable of privately addressing their conflicts, they are good candidates. However, in the cases where there are extensive unaddressed issues in a relationship, a couple may benefit more from counseling rather than this form of a couples' group that focuses on enrichment, run by lay leaders; **it is critical to be clear that this is not a therapy group.** A fundamental agreement is that if these conversations reveal issues that require professional attention, the leaders will kindly suggest to the couple that they seek counseling. The needs of one couple should not take over your group.

Considerations Regarding Age

Time of Day: People in the winter season of their lives often find it difficult to attend meetings at night due to visual impairment, so you may want to schedule your meetings in the afternoons or mornings when there is enough daylight. At your first meeting, the group can discuss when, where, and for how long they wish to meet.

Setting & Hearing Issues: Choose a quiet, warm, friendly, protected space to meet. It is common for elders to suffer from hearing and visual decline. If you don't address these issues (with microphones, for instance, or a small enough room), those who can't hear will drop out or get frustrated, as it is painful and isolating to not be able to follow what is going on. If you are showing videos, use closed captions. The Touchstones ensure that only one person speaks at a time, which helps address hearing loss issues by reducing multiple conversations. However, when people share in a vulnerable manner, their voices tend to drop. If this is a problem, you can use a microphone that can be passed around to each speaker. In other words, do all you can do for the people who can't hear well to ensure they have a positive experience.

Visual Challenges: For individuals with visual problems, they may read the book on an e-book reader, where they can use a larger font. If you provide printed materials, use a clear font in at least 14-point size, and double space, so it is easier to read.

Common Physical Challenges: Individuals with back issues may have problems sitting for long periods of time, so frequent breaks, comfortable seating, and shortened sessions can all help. Invite people with back issues to bring a special chair or whatever it will take for them to attend. It will be up to the leader to check in with the group and make appropriate adjustments.

For Individuals Experiencing Dementia: Finally, and sadly, if someone in a couple is suffering from a serious form of dementia, participation in this group is inappropriate. To create a safe space, participants need to be capable of learning the rules, following the boundaries as outlined in the

Touchstones when others share, and being able to discuss the reading. While a painful reality to name and enforce, you are protecting them and the group as well. In this situation, encourage the couple to seek out a support group for individuals suffering from dementia.

Attendance

To ensure continuity, it's highly recommended that group members commit to faithful attendance at all of the meetings to the best of their ability. Trust builds over time, and poor attendance, leaving the meetings early, or arriving late undermines this trust and interweaving of group connections. Of course, legitimate interruptions occur, and there is always room for extending grace for understandable absences. It would be wise to inform the couples in writing about these expectations, including the agreements to attend the meetings regularly, read the chapters in advance of each meeting, and respect and adhere to the Touchstones.

Overview of What Happens in a Meeting

Choose one chapter for your focus per meeting and request that **it be read before attending** as these chapters are too long to read aloud. It is a good idea to write an email to the group reminding them of what chapter to read and when the meeting is to occur. Upon arrival, you can welcome the group and begin the session by asking participants how they have been living with the themes in the program since you last met. Ask the group, "Are there any questions, insights, or stories you wish to share with each other before diving into this next chapter?" To refresh the group about the chapter to be discussed, you can show the couple's video interview excerpt at www.sidebysideaging.com or give an oral summary of their marriage story. Then allow at least twenty minutes for silent reflection and journaling based on the questions provided in this guide for that chapter. Encourage the participants to choose the questions that speak to them or write their own questions if they wish. Since this is a soulful process, less is more. The timing should always feel relaxed and not rushed, with space for welcoming silence when no one is sharing. As the group leader, you always participate. You are encouraged to add your own touches, which may include poetry, music, beautiful centerpieces, YouTube clips, and rituals that fit your leadership style and the group you serve. Finally, suggest that the couples continue to extend the learning by reflecting at home on the questions you did not have time to address in the group.

What to Bring to Each Session

We recommend that participants bring a journal, pen, and a copy of *Side by Side*. If anyone misses a session, they can do the work at home since the reflection questions are embedded in the guide.

Touchstones for Creating Safe Space

When we participate in a group with the goals of personal or spiritual reflection, we enter into a covenant with each other to be faithful to how we listen, share, and, most importantly, hold what is disclosed in confidence. Based on our twenty-five years of work through the Center for Courage & Renewal facilitating the Circle of Trust approach, we recommend using the Touchstones (appendix II), which serve as the "rules of engagement" for your group. Take turns reading each Touchstone aloud at the beginning of every meeting (not just the first session). If something goes wrong in your group interactions, ask, "What touchstone did we violate or not follow?" Or "I'd like to lift up this touchstone again as a reminder of how we've agreed to interact," and then try not to make the same mistake again.

The Touchstones are powerful practices for interacting with others, and can even become new practices for couples at home.

Group Sharing

Circles of Trust move from solo reflection to dyad/small-group sharing to large-group reflection, often with suggested prompts. After giving time for individual reflection, the leader invites whoever wishes to speak into the small circle. Sharing is always optional and never mandated. Individuals can choose to listen and not talk about their writing (as stated in the touchstone, "This is not share or die"). Unlike other groups, we never go around the circle and demand that someone speaks, but instead, we allow people to speak if and when they feel ready. The leader makes sure that everyone who wishes gets a chance to share. The leader can speak first to break the silence if necessary and model what is being asked of participants. If someone goes on too long, gently say, "We need to move on so everyone gets a chance to speak."

When an Individual Speaks

In this format, we listen respectfully and do not comment on or debate what another person says (that's where the "turning to wonder" and "speak with an 'I' statement" touchstones come in). Unlike a traditional book group, this sharing comes from a personal response, which is never debated. The point is not to question or judge anything about the couples as portrayed in their chapter but to reflect on what comes up for you in your own life and relationship. There is no "right or wrong" response to any prompt, but only each person's truth or story about what they hear in the chapter or in their reflections. We never comment on what someone else reveals in a dyad or small group but speak for ourselves. If this guideline is violated, the group will quickly become unsafe, and the sharing will remain on the surface.

The Closing Circle

Once everyone who wishes to do so has shared their reflections, the leader will end the meeting with a closing circle. This allows the participants to state briefly what insights or surprises they experienced while reading and reflecting on a chapter or while listening to one another. To end the circle, ask someone to read aloud the "Beatitudes for Couples," or for multiple-session groups, end with the one beatitude and/or epigraph that goes with the chapter discussed—we call this a "grace note."

A SAMPLE AGENDA

Below is a simple format for structuring a *Side by Side* group process based on a two-hour meeting.

2:00–2:20 (20 min.) Welcome & Check-in

The leader welcomes the group and invites a brief check-in before reflecting on the chapter for this session. You might ask questions like, "How has this work been living in you since we last met? What questions, stories, or insights from our work last week would you like to share?" or, "What beatitude or touchstone is speaking to you at this time?"

Regarding the first session: In advance, be sure the group has read the introduction and first chapter of *Side by Side*. For the first session, begin by asking people to introduce themselves and share why they joined the group and what questions they carry regarding the themes found in *Side by Side*: aging, spirituality, and relationships.

Caution: Be careful, or this check-in can use up lots of time. If you find this portion valuable, you can extend the group's time to two-and-a-half hours or gather for a soup supper and check in before the official session begins.

2:20–2:25 (5 min.) *Touchstones*

At each meeting, take turns reading the Touchstones aloud to reinforce your group agreements. If you wish, discuss them and how they might be speaking to you or challenging you, both in this group or in your personal lives and relationships.

2:25–2:30 (5 min.) *Refreshing the Story*

Whether or not the participants have read the chapter in advance, as leader you can share the chapter-couple's video excerpt and/or summarize the themes and essence of the couple's marriage story, then ask participants to briefly say what spoke to, disturbed, resonated, or amused them.

2:30–2:50 (20 min.) *A Time for Solo Reflection (and bio break if needed)*

Invite the group, in silence, to write in their journals for fifteen to twenty minutes in response to one or more of the questions for this chapter. Participants can choose from these questions or write their own. Some may want to draw images, make a list of thoughts, or sit and enjoy silent reflection during this time. Not everyone likes to write. If the group ends writing earlier than twenty minutes, you can begin the sharing early. Finally, you will probably have people who haven't done the reading. They will have to answer the questions without the advantage of the couple's chapter informing them.

Built-In Break: Note that five minutes is built into the solo period as a bio-break. Make sure it doesn't turn into run-away socializing by requesting that silence be maintained.

2:50–3:20 (30 min.) Dyad/Small Group Sharing

For this half hour, the group leader has many choices for structuring the sharing from the journaling/solo reflections. Couples can turn to each other and discuss what they have written about. At times, you may wish to invite two couples to meet as a group of four. You can also stay in the large group or invite couples to go on a "walk and talk" with each other, taking turns listening and talking, with fifteen minutes for each person to share while the partner simply listens.

3:20–3:40 (20 min.) Large Group Sharing

Bring the group back together and invite anyone who wishes to discuss what they have learned during the smaller group session. At times, you might ask people to journal for five minutes to collect their thoughts before sharing in the large group.

3:45–4:00 (15 min.) Closing Circle & Grace Note

To end, invite anyone who wishes to briefly state, in a sentence or two, what has touched them during this time, an insight they are taking away from the group, or simply how they are feeling. As a Grace Note to end the meeting, the group reads aloud one or more of the "Beatitudes for Couples," or the epigraph (quote) that ended the chapter, or any other short quote, song, or poem that delights and inspires you.

Homework: Before leaving the session, be sure to remind participants of the date and time for the next meeting, and the next chapter reading assignment, as well as a "homework" suggestion to continue exploring the questions and practices that go with this session. There is more to each chapter than can be addressed within the time limits of a single group session. Those who want to go deeper can do so in between meetings by journaling, discussing, and reflecting on stories and questions in this guide. If the group wants to schedule another meeting on the same chapter, that is fine. The soul thrives with more time for reflection.

A Grace Note of Gratitude for the Leader: Choosing to organize a couples' group is a generous gift to your community that entails your time, your experience and skills, and your commitment. If you wish to gain more background in the Circle of Trust approach, visit the Center for Courage & Renewal website, www.couragerenewal.org, to learn about retreats and offerings that teach people about the nuances and philosophy of this process. If you haven't done so, we strongly recommend reading *A Hidden Wholeness: The Journey Toward an Undivided Life* by Parker J. Palmer. In this book, the author outlines how and why we hold space for the community in the ways of Circles of Trust, providing more detail than is possible in this guide. Finally, the authors will be offering retreats and further support and resources for organizing *Side by Side* couples' groups, which will be posted on their website: www.sidebysideaging.com. You may contact the authors through this website as well.

REFLECTION QUESTIONS FOR EACH CHAPTER
Chapter 1: Blessed Is the Couple Who Welcomes Divine Presence into Their Midst
JIM & MARIANNE HOUSTON

1. *Blessed is the couple who welcomes Divine Presence into their midst, for they shall know Eternal Belonging, grace, and love* is the beatitude that frames Jim and Marianne's story. How does this beatitude speak to you as a couple? How do you welcome Divine Presence into your relationship?
2. Which of their stories speaks to you, and why?
3. Recount an early memory of a spiritual experience.
4. How has your faith journey unfolded over time?

5. If your photos could talk, what stories would they reveal about each of your family of origin cultures, races, and religious backgrounds, and how you have brought them together?
6. Jim and Marianne were pioneers in terms of entering a racially mixed marriage. Is there an area in your relationship where you have been pioneers?
7. If communication is the daily bread of relationships, in what ways and with what rules were you each raised in terms of communication styles that impact your encounters? How have they played out in your relationship?
8. In terms of raising children, did you experience tensions related to different values and practices? How have you addressed these differences? Now that your children are adults, what has changed in your parenting with them?
9. In regards to extroversion/introversion, where do you each land, and how has this influenced your relationship over time?
10. Where in your life are you able to interact with young people? What do you give and receive in these relationships?
11. At this time of life, in what ways are you turning your service work towards home, if at all?
12. What elders have you known who are models for aging? Write a tribute to one of them.
13. If you could sit down to dinner with Jim and Marianne, what topics would you like to talk about with them?

Chapter 2: Blessed Is the Couple Who Embraces All Seasons of Life
CARYL & JEFF CRESWELL

1. *Blessed is the couple who embraces all seasons of life—the perennial cycles of spring, summer, autumn,*

and winter—for they shall know wholeness is the beatitude for Caryl and Jeff. How does this beatitude speak to you as a couple or not? What season are you in at this time in your relationship?

2. What is the nature of your commitment or the vows you made with each other as a couple? In practice, what has most helped you "stick it out" through the dark times?
3. In what ways have you supported each other in integrating your "souls and roles" in order for you each to fulfill your life purpose? How are you similar and different in relation to this topic?
4. As a couple or as an individual, how do you discern what is important to you? What discernment practices do you employ?
5. Discuss ways you are "caretaking" for each other. What discussions have you had about how to care for one another and what your wishes are for future developments in your health?
6. Imagine what it would look like to respect each other's dignity in the process of taking care of each other. What comes to mind? What would you want and need when receiving care?
7. What does this couple have to say about supporting friends through loss and widowhood? What do you want to remember and practice from their suggestions?
8. Consider the "Four Wondering Questions" from Godly Play, and take some time to answer them together daily for a week. Can you imagine using these each evening as a way of staying current with each other, and yourselves? Would you change them, or add to them?

The Four Wondering Questions:
What was the best part of the day?
What was the most important part of the day?

What was just for you?
What could you have left out?
9. If you could have dinner with Caryl & Jeff, what topics, stories, or questions would you like to address with them?

Chapter 3: Blessed Is the Couple Who Welcomes the Stranger
LAURIE RUTENBERG & GARY SCHOENBERG

1. *Blessed is the couple who welcomes the stranger in each other, for they shall find wonder and encouragement on their growing edges* is the beatitude for Gary and Laurie. How does this speak to you?
2. In what ways have you become strangers to one another? Have you undergone long periods of estrangement? What creates estrangement and distance in your relationship?
3. How have you learned to cross the Gesher (footbridge) of your differences and times of estrangement in ways that bring you closer? What behaviors or attitudes have you observed that take you farther apart?
4. In your years together, what questions have become quests you have held over time? What questions are you holding now about your aging or life? Your relationship? Your spirituality?
5. In what ways do you invite the Sabbath to "keep you?" Where does Sabbath live in your lives, alone and together—i.e. creating time for silence, breaking bread, telling stories, being in nature, blessing your children, slowing down, and practicing devotion?
6. What do you want to say to your children about your death and your wishes for end-of-life care? What messages do you want to give your children about death?

7. If you could sit down for a Shabbat meal with the rabbis, what would you want to ask them? What stories would you share with them?

Longer Activities: The following suggestions will take longer to accomplish than you will have time for in the group. You can try them at home in the coming weeks before your next group session.

A. Write a Teshuvah letter to one another, as described by the rabbis, and then light a candle, turn off the phones and computers, and read them aloud to each other. If you wish, then write Teshuvah letters to your children. (If you haven't read this chapter, you can find the description of a Teshuvah letter within it.)

B. Write the stories of your parents' deaths in great detail. When done, take turns reading them aloud. Listen to how their deaths have become teachers to you.

C. Write a living will, or a legacy statement identifying what qualities and values you hope to bequeath to the people you care about when you depart from this world.

Chapter 4: Blessed Is the Couple Who Confronts Their Own Shadows
PAUL & ROZ DUMESNIL

1. *Blessed is the couple who confronts their own shadows, for they shall be freed from blame and projection* is the beatitude for this couple. How does it speak to your experience?

2. When you notice an appearance of a shadow quality you are casting on your partner, how do you generally behave? Can you think of an example? Consider naming the reoccurring shadows that seem to haunt your relationship.

3. In your relationship, what does "going to the mat together" mean to you? What does it actually look like? Think about the times you have done so in your relationship that stand out.
4. How would you describe your repair process when you experience a breakdown in your relationship? When you hurt each other, how do you mend your relationship? When was the last time you had to do so?
5. As you reflect on your relationship (or lack thereof) with churches and other spiritual communities, what have been your experiences? What have you gained from them? How have they been problematic or life-giving?
6. Like Roz and Paul, have you noticed more of a draw toward your inner life and contemplative practices as you age? A slower pace? A need for more solitude, silence, journaling, reading, or time in nature? How are you similar or different in these areas? What sort of atmosphere do you create in your home?
7. In what ways must you "honor your limits" at this time? How has that impacted how you live together as a couple?
8. When you consider the illnesses you have encountered so far, how might you read them symbolically? Have you witnessed in one another how health challenges have built character?
9. Has your experience with the dying verified the saying, "You die as you live?" How do Roz's final words speak to you? What do you hope your final words will be?
10. How do you "keep death before you," or experience mini-deaths and resurrections while still alive? At this age, with "the end in sight," how does this impact how you live today?
11. If you could share dinner with Paul and Roz, what would you like to talk about?

***Chapter 5: Blessed Is the Couple Who
Listens Deeply to Each Other***
STEVE & FAYE ORTON SNYDER

1. *Blessed is the couple who listens deeply to each other, for they shall be seen, understood, and met* is the beatitude for this couple. When you consider your listening to one another with your minds, bodies, hearts, and souls, how is it going? Where might you improve?
2. What values do you consider to be the bedrock of your relationship? Perhaps you have made them explicit as commitments, agreements, or vows. How do you know when you have digressed from these values? And what do you do?
3. How do you seek and find support for your relationship when you come across roadblocks and troubles that are bigger than the two of you? To whom do you turn for help?
4. From reading about the "geography of loss" in Steve and Faye's lives, what are your takeaways from their experiences that inform your relationship? What is your collective "geography of loss" as a couple?
5. How have you learned to carry loss? What list of names would be in your wallet?
6. Take time to share with one another about when you feel most loved in your relationship. What small gestures and other ways of being communicate love, nurturing, and care?
7. What activities no longer hold meaning for you that, in the past, were an important focus? What is taking their place?
8. If you could sit down for a meal with Faye and Steve, what would you like to discuss with them?

Chapter 6: Blessed Is the Couple Who
Practices Compassion
BOBBY BELLAMY & BARBARA BLAIN-BELLAMY

1. *Blessed is the couple who practices compassion, for they shall honor the Spark of the Divine in all of their brothers and sisters* is the beatitude for this couple. Where in your relationship are you most in need of compassion at this time?
2. As you reflect on your relationship, ask, "In what ways are we a home to one another?"
3. If you saw every person you met as if they were Jesus or a beloved child of God, how would this change your relationships?
4. Barbara names the inner quality of judging others as interfering with her practice of treating people with compassion. What inner quality gets in your way of loving others or interferes with your love as a couple?
5. Barbara and Bobby share many beliefs and practices related to their Christianity, including the belief in the goodness of God, following the Commandments, praying, tithing, and forgiving. What spiritual beliefs do you share as a couple? How have these beliefs manifested as practices in your relationship?
6. Recall any mystical incidents either of you has experienced. How have they influenced your spiritual journeys?
7. What statements can you make and stand by about love at this time in life?
8. If you could have dinner with Barbara and Bobby, what would you like to discuss with them?

Chapter 7: Blessed Is the Couple Who
Enjoys the Fruits of Mutuality
SALLY HARE & JIM ROGERS

1. *Blessed is the couple who cares about the other's needs as much as their own, for they shall enjoy the fruits*

of mutuality is the beatitude for this couple. What place does mutuality hold in your relationship? Think of some examples of when you have practiced mutuality in your life choices together.
2. When you consider your own experiences with inherited gender roles, what has transpired over time in your relationship?
3. Reflect on your parents' relationships, and discuss how you have followed some of the same paths and where you may have diverged and changed.
4. What are your hopes for your children's relationships and lives? If they asked, what would you share with them about parenting? Life? Gender roles? Marriage?
5. What does looking at your own and each other's aging "with soft eyes" mean to you?
6. Name the rigors and gifts of aging you are undergoing at this time.
7. If you were blessed with being at your parents' sides when they died, what did you learn from them? What regrets do you have? How do you continue to honor them?
8. In these difficult times of climate change, social, and political unrest, what are you outraged about, and how do you see yourselves addressing these issues now?
9. If you could have dinner with Sally and Jim, what would you want to talk about?

Chapter 8: Blessed Is the Couple Who Extends Tender Care When Suffering
ANNE & TOM BUTLER

1. *Blessed is the couple who extends tender care to one another when suffering, diminished, wounded, or shamed, for they shall be comforted* is the beatitude for this couple. As you read about Anne and Tom's

relationship, ask, "What does tender care mean to us? In what ways do we express it to each other?"
2. What story spoke to you when reading this chapter?
3. Has there been an "Abraham" moment in your life regarding your relationship? What did you have to give up or leave behind in order to be together?
4. In what ways were you a "foreign country" to one another, bringing together your personalities?
5. What significant transitions have you undergone in your relationship?
6. Has there been a time when what disturbed you also nourished you?
7. Anne quotes Richard Rohr as saying pain that is not transformed is transmitted. Think of a recent time when you faced a difficult situation and "transformed" it. Or one you ignored, and what happened as a result. Is there an issue now that could use transformation and your tender attention?
8. Where do you find conditions for hospitality, sanctuary, and respite as a couple? In what ways do you offer them to others?
9. From Anne and Tom's stories regarding inviting Spirit into their conflicts, what wisdom, if any, do you glean for your relationship?
10. In what ways have you experienced, addressed, and tended to each other's family of origin wounds and trauma? How have you helped each other? What have you learned in the process? How has Spirit entered into these tender places?
11. What regular spiritual practices (like the Butlers' use of John O'Donohue's poem "A Mirror of Questions" from *To Bless the Space Between Us*) have you put into place to enhance and deepen your relationship? If you wish, practice these

questions this week, and see if they work for you. Below are examples of two of the questions similar to the ones in his book, and/or you may want to craft your own. (For the full list of questions, see page 98 in *To Bless the Space Between Us*.)
- Where did I feel the pain of a wound today, and no one noticed?
- I wonder why I was given this day.

12. If you could have dinner with Anne and Tom, what would you like to discuss with them?

Chapter 9: Blessed Is the Couple Who Recognizes the Indwelling Spirit in All of Life
PATSY GRACE & HARVEY BOTTELSEN

1. *Blessed is the couple who recognizes the Indwelling Spirit in all of life, for they shall encounter the Mystery and see the Light in all beings* is the beatitude for this couple. How does this beatitude speak to you? Think of an experience when this beatitude came alive for you.
2. Patsy and Harvey's home is filled with crystals. If we walked into your home to interview you, what artifacts would we notice surrounding you that reflect the essence of your relationship?
3. Recall your first meeting and what you saw in each other. Was there a "soul recognition" at the time?
4. Was there anything about your beginnings that suggested the path or trajectory you would follow as a couple?
5. Is there a spiritual teacher or tradition at the center of your relationship around which much of your lives organize? What are the central teachings of this teacher?
6. Is there a word like Patsy and Harvey's word, "enchantment," that captures the nature of your spirituality, and how you live?

7. Looking back over your relationship, what was your most challenging incident? Have you gone through a period of separation? How did you work through it? What did you learn?
8. Have there been medical challenges that have led you to a deeper understanding of your interdependence?
9. If you have children, what would you like them to say about you at your funeral?
10. If you could sit down to dinner with Patsy and Harvey, what topics or questions would you like to entertain with them?

Chapter 10: Blessed Is the Couple Who Dances with the Tension Between "Me" & "We"
RICK & MARCY JACKSON

1. *Blessed is the couple who dances with the tension between "me" and "we," for they shall know companioning without loss of self* is the beatitude for this couple. In regards to the tension between "me" and "we," what comes to mind when you reflect on your relationship?
2. Considering your history, were there times in your relationship when you felt you lost yourself? What happened? How did you regain your footing and differentiation?
3. Have there been times when you felt like you were living parallel lives, out of touch with each other, and too focused on your own goals and activities? What does age ask of you now regarding this dance of "me" and "we"?
4. What unspoken assumptions and expectations did you bring into your relationship?
5. When or have you run into gender role expectations in your relationship? How or have they changed with time?
6. In what ways have you learned to mirror each other's shadows and become "truth tellers" for each other?

7. In terms of the theme of "soul and role," what commitments, interests, and creative endeavors are calling you now? What is naturally ending, and what is bringing you alive that is fresh and new?
8. If you have adult children, what have you learned about being in a healthy, life-giving relationship with them? What are the possibilities and limits in your relationship with your children?
9. If you could have dinner with the Jacksons, what would you wish to talk about?

Chapter 11: Blessed Is the Couple Who Practices Sabbath
KAREN NOORDHOFF & DAVID HAGSTROM

1. *Blessed is the couple who practices Sabbath through the daily bread of devotion, mindfulness, and prayer, for they shall find Home* is the beatitude for this couple. David and Karen described how each evening they "observe the Sabbath" or take time to rest, enjoy a glass of wine, share spiritual readings, and pray. Consider your relationship and how you already or may want to "observe the Sabbath" or create a sanctuary for reflection and prayer together.
2. When you think about the notion of mutuality and sacrificing your own needs for your partner in your relationship, does a story comes to mind where you practiced it, like when David left Alaska? How do you discern when it is time for you to offer your partner this gift of putting their needs on the front burner?
3. Love is often expressed without words and has a lot to do with attunement with your partner. Take some time to spell out some of the qualities of your attunement with each other that capture your relationship at this stage of life. Consider how your love has been flavored with time, maturity, and a shared history.

4. David stated, "The adventure now is about growing older together." When you look at aging together as an adventure, what does this mean to you? How might you improve or enhance this adventure?
5. If there is an age difference in your relationship, share with each other what your experience with it is like.
6. Jean Vanier names a new "freedom from function" with aging. Karen and David focus on their creativity and writing lives with this new freedom. How about you?
7. In what ways do you "pull down the shades" for yourselves as a couple? When do you find it necessary?
8. Are there experiences about which you tell fundamentally different stories, like their different stories about leaving Alaska?
9. Couples tend to be drawn to certain landscapes and countries like Karen and David's affinity for Alaska and France. As you reflect on your lives, which adventures and places have helped define you?
10. Karen and David claim that "slow time" is a way they move in the world. How would you name your timing and relationship with time as a couple?
11. If you could share a meal with Karen and David, what would you like to discuss with them?

Chapter 12: Blessed Is the Couple Who Extends Mercy and Forgiveness
MICHAEL & EILEEN HEATON

1. *Blessed is the couple who extends mercy and forgiveness, for they shall be relieved of resentment and harsh judgment* is the beatitude for this couple. When have you been called to extend mercy to one another in small and large ways?
2. Michael and Eileen deeply admire and respect each other. Take some time to share what you admire and

cherish about your partner. Ask: Do we tell each other often enough how much we appreciate each other?
3. Describe how you assist one another by mirroring back what you are seeing. What are the best conditions for both offering and receiving mirroring? How open are you to receiving mirroring? How do you deflect it?
4. What is the difference between mercy and forgiveness, according to Eileen? Does this distinction speak to you? Can you think of a time when mercy was more appropriate than forgiveness?
5. How would you describe your forgiveness process? Does a story come to mind where you needed to extend forgiveness to each other in your relationship?
6. What "tools," like the Enneagram or the Myers-Briggs Type Indicator, have assisted your growth as a couple? Could you use some now?
7. How does being in this stage of life, as "Forest Dwellers," speak to you? Where are you on this continuum of life, as defined in Hinduism?
8. If you could share dinner with Eileen and Michael, what would you like to talk about?

Chapter 13: Blessed Is the Couple Who Offers Beneficial Presence Across the Generations
RUTH SHAGOURY & JIM WHITNEY

1. *Blessed is the couple who offers beneficial presence across the generations, for they shall leave a legacy of love* is the beatitude for this couple. When you reflect on the notion of beneficial presence across the generations, what examples come to mind with the couples you know?
2. What place do play and tomfoolery take in your lives? Can you imagine increasing them as a couple? Where is the fun in your relationship?

3. Ruth names the time when Jim put her PJs in the dryer for her after a long day of teaching as a symbol of his thoughtful caring and support; she keeps track of the good things he does for her. Name some incidents where your partner showed care for you in a special way. This week, consider keeping track of the kind, thoughtful gestures you extend to one another.
4. In what ways have you created structures for your days, post-retirement? As a couple, what advantages and challenges have you encountered regarding spending more time together?
5. When you think of the concept of your "unlived life," what comes to mind? What new creative endeavors or activities do you find yourselves trying out where you are not experts but beginners? Have you picked up or re-upped interests you didn't have time to cultivate earlier in life?
6. If you were to prepare a dish that represented creativity to you as a couple, what would it be?
7. The German phrase "Jugend und ältesten, austausch zwischen" means the intense, beneficial exchange between youth and elders, an expression that recognizes the energy transference from one generation to the other. Do you enjoy such relationships at this time? Whom did you know throughout your childhoods who offered you this beneficial generational exchange?
8. Jim and Ruth hold a strong belief system about how to care for aging parents. How did you respond to their approach, and what are your thoughts about the "right practices" in caring for the elderly? In what spirit would you like to be held when or if you get in the position of needing such care?
9. What, if any, conversations have you had with your children regarding your aging and the potential need for their care?

10. When you read "The generations are important to each other," what comes to mind from your experience?
11. If you could enjoy dinner with Jim and Ruth, what would you want to discuss with them?

ADDITIONAL PRACTICES & ACTIVITIES FOR *SIDE BY SIDE*

Interview Each Other

Invite one couple to interview another couple using the questions in appendix I. Our original interviews took up to six hours, so your interviews may require ongoing meetings. Or, if you wish to recreate the conditions we enjoyed, spend a weekend together for the interview process. If you have a camera, videotape the interview and give it to the couple, or record it on a phone. If you are close to your children, ask them to conduct the interview; they will learn a lot about you too.

Create a Recommitment Ceremony

Invite the married couples to locate their original ceremony and vows if possible. Then craft a recommitment ceremony that reflects their relationship today. Ask a friend or your minister/rabbi/priest to officiate for you. Commitment ceremonies usually involve some of the following:

- Invocation or opening prayer
- Favorite music (a song that captures your love and the nature of your relationship)
- One or more readings or poems
- Comments by the officiant about relationships and the nature of commitment
- Exchange of vows
- Exchange of rings
- Final blessing

Write Your Own Beatitudes or Touchstones

Write beatitudes or touchstones for your relationship that best suit you, or edit the existing list in your own words.

Create a Film Series or Book Group with Friends

Invite a group of friends to form a film or book study group, and then take turns choosing films or books that address relationships, aging, or spirituality. We'd love to hear what you come up with! Post your findings on our website.

Relationship Enlightenment & Adventure Pilgrimages

Plan a trip focusing on "relationship enlightenment and adventure" where you visit the places and people that have held the most meaning for you over the years and perhaps the site where you got married. You could travel to the places where you were born and raised and revisit your favorite hikes or spots in nature, cities, or countries. Undergo a spiritual pilgrimage to a sacred site representing your faith tradition, such as walking the Camino or spending a week in silence. Create questions you wish to travel with you, and integrate regular times for journaling, reflection, and prayer. Draw a map of where you will travel to, and if you are unable to actually go on a trip, enjoy the process and memories involved in the planning.

Finally, time spent in silence can be very nurturing for a relationship. Agree to spend a weekend at home, at a cabin, or a retreat center in complete silence, and then share your experiences with each other.

Notes

INTRODUCTION

1. Rinker Buck, *The Oregon Trail: An American Journey*, (New York: Simon & Shuster, 2015), 1.
2. "Soul Stories versus Ego Stories" is an idea created by Courage & Renewal facilitators Marcy Jackson and Parker J. Palmer for use in Circle of Trust retreats and is included with their permission.

CHAPTER 2 CARYL & JEFF CRESWELL

1. "The Four Wondering Questions" are from the Godly Play Foundation, created for programs that nurture children's spirituality. See https://godlyplayfoundation.org.

CHAPTER 3 LAURIE RUTENBERG & GARY SCHOENBERG

1. Many of the stories in this chapter about Rabbi Laurie Rutenberg and Rabbi Gary Schoenberg have previously appeared in other publications, including *Gesher: A Journal of Outreach and Welcome* and *Gesher: A Bridge Home*, published from 1993 to 2003; their unpublished manuscript entitled *River of Souls: Guiding Jewish Americans' Home*; and many articles, including, "A New Kind of Rabbinate: Reaching Out to Unaffiliated Jews," Laurie Rutenberg, *CCAR Journal: A Reform Jewish Quarterly* (1997). To learn more about their work, request a preview of *River of Souls*, or access their *Gesher Journal* archives, visit https://ourjewishhome.org/.

CHAPTER 4 PAUL & ROZ DUMESNIL

1 James Hillman, *The Force of Character: And the Lasting Life* (New York: Ballantine Books, 2000), 58.

CHAPTER 7 SALLY HARE & JIM ROGERS

1 A clearness committee is a Quaker practice of discernment that is a key part of the Circle of Trust approach by the Center for Courage & Renewal. Sally Hare is one of the founding facilitators to develop this approach and the related Touchstones. See an article by Parker J. Palmer at https://couragerenewal.org/library/the-clearness-committee-a-communal-approach-to-discernment/.

CHAPTER 8 ANNE & TOM BUTLER

1 Mary Catherine Bateson, "Living as an Improvisational Art" October 1, 2015, in On Being, hosted by Krista Tippett, podcast, MP3 audio, 50:03, https://onbeing.org/programs/mary-catherine-bateson-living-as-an-improvisational-art/.

2 John O'Donohue, *To Bless the Space Between Us: A Book of Blessings* (New York: Doubleday, 2008), 98.

CHAPTER 9 PATSY GRACE & HARVEY BOTTELSEN

1 Richard Rohr, *The Universal Christ: How a Forgotten Reality Can Change Everything We See, Hope For, and Believe* (New York: Convergent Books, 2019); see also Brie Stoner and Paul Swanson, "Universal Christ Values (Part I)," February 15, 2020, in *Another Name for Every Thing with Richard Rohr*, hosted by Richard Rohr, podcast, MP3 audio, 60:15, https://cac.org/podcasts/universal-christ-values-part-1/.

2 The Five Wishes Advance Care Planning: https://fivewishes.org.

3 Stephen Cope, *The Great Work of Your Life: A Guide for the Journey to Your True Calling* (New York: Bantam Books, 2012), 53.

4 Robert A. Johnson and Jerry M. Ruhl, *Living Your Unlived Life: Coping with Unrealized Dreams and Fulfilling Your Purpose in the Second Half of Life* (New York: Jeremy Tarcher/Penguin Publishers, 2007), 23.

CHAPTER 10 RICK & MARCY JACKSON

1 "Warriors for the Human Spirit: Training to be the Presence of Insight and Compassion," Margaret Wheatley's official website, accessed April 18, 2023, https://margaretwheatley.com/2020-europe-warriors-for-the-human-spirit-training/.

CHAPTER 11 KAREN NOORDHOFF & DAVID HAGSTROM

1 Jean Vanier, *Community and Growth* (Mahwah, NJ: Paulist Press, 1989).

2 David Hagstrom, *Messengers of Encouragement: Stories to Help Us Listen, Support and Believe in One Another* (Bend, OR: Dancing Moon Press, 2021).

3 Joyce Rupp, *Boundless Compassion: Creating a Way of Life* (Notre Dame, IN: Sorin Books, 2018).

CHAPTER 13 RUTH SHAGOURY & JIM WHITNEY

1 Robert A. Johnson and Jerry M. Ruhl, *Living Your Unlived Life: Coping with Unrealized Dreams and Fulfilling Your Purpose in the Second Half of Life* (New York: Jeremy Tarcher/Penguin Publishers, 2007), 14.

2 Ruth Shagoury, "My Mother's Hands" (unpublished personal journal entry, October 2013), used by permission of the author.

CONCLUSION

1 Terrence Real, *The New Rules of Marriage: What You Need to Know to Make Love Work* (New York: Ballantine Books, 2007).

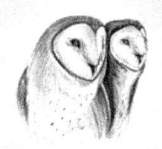

Deepen Your Journey

The authors are available for speaking engagements, book club talks, retreats and workshops, and consulting. For small-group resources to supplement the Readers' Guide, including video clips, visit www.sidebysideaging.com.

About the Authors

Caryl Casbon is a poet, writer, and author of *The Everywhere Oracle: A Guided Journey Through Poetry for an Ensouled World* (Wyatt-MacKenzie Publishing, 2015.) A facilitator through the Center for Courage & Renewal, she has co-written programs dedicated to exploring the inner life, including A Geography of Grace, Befriending the Unknown, The Soul of Aging, and The Anamcara Project and Storybook. She also works as an interfaith minister and spiritual director and has led retreats for over twenty-five years.

Jay Casbon retired in 2016 from Oregon State University as the first provost of the new Bend Campus for Oregon State University after a lifetime of leadership and teaching in higher education, including thirteen years at Lewis & Clark College as dean of graduate studies. Jay also worked internationally in Ecuador, Peru, China, Germany, Austria, and Italy. Throughout his academic tenure, he published numerous scholarly articles. Currently, Jay serves as a consultant for universities addressing the need for redesign.

Married since 2001, Caryl and Jay live in Santa Barbara, California. They offer extended learning opportunities for working with couples' groups, online seminars, and in-person retreats. They are both Circle of Trust® facilitators prepared by the Center for Courage & Renewal. Contact the Casbons at www.sidebysideaging.com.

About Creative Courage Press

CREATIVE COURAGE PRESS is a small, independent publishing company founded in 2020 by Shelly L. Francis, inspired by the people she met while writing *The Courage Way: Leading and Living with Integrity* (Berrett-Koehler, 2018). Now, in collaboration with other authors, we are creating courage for the complexity of being human.

Get to know the essential voices of our remarkable authors and their refreshing ideas for leading change from the heart. Together we hope to generate meaningful conversations in our communities.

Visit us online to get fortified with resources and reflections for creating your own courageous way of life. As we grow, we invite you to grow with us.

www.CreativeCouragePress.com
hello@CreativeCouragePress.com

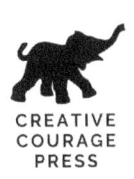

CREATIVE
COURAGE
PRESS

Printed in the USA
CPSIA information can be obtained
at www.ICGtesting.com
BVHW030042280823
668896BV00003B/17